Eva-Luise Hobl

Methotrexate in Rheumatoid Arthritis

Eva-Luise Hobl

Methotrexate in Rheumatoid Arthritis

A pharmacokinetic-pharmacodynamic-pharmacogenomic Model

Südwestdeutscher Verlag für Hochschulschriften

Impressum/Imprint (nur für Deutschland/only for Germany)
Bibliografische Information der Deutschen Nationalbibliothek: Die Deutsche Nationalbibliothek verzeichnet diese Publikation in der Deutschen Nationalbibliografie; detaillierte bibliografische Daten sind im Internet über http://dnb.d-nb.de abrufbar.
Alle in diesem Buch genannten Marken und Produktnamen unterliegen warenzeichen-, marken- oder patentrechtlichem Schutz bzw. sind Warenzeichen oder eingetragene Warenzeichen der jeweiligen Inhaber. Die Wiedergabe von Marken, Produktnamen, Gebrauchsnamen, Handelsnamen, Warenbezeichnungen u.s.w. in diesem Werk berechtigt auch ohne besondere Kennzeichnung nicht zu der Annahme, dass solche Namen im Sinne der Warenzeichen- und Markenschutzgesetzgebung als frei zu betrachten wären und daher von jedermann benutzt werden dürften.

Coverbild: www.ingimage.com

Verlag: Südwestdeutscher Verlag für Hochschulschriften GmbH & Co. KG
Heinrich-Böcking-Str. 6-8, 66121 Saarbrücken, Deutschland
Telefon +49 681 37 20 271-1, Telefax +49 681 37 20 271-0
Email: info@svh-verlag.de

Zugl.: Vienna, Medical University of Vienna, Diss., 2011

Herstellung in Deutschland (siehe letzte Seite)
ISBN: 978-3-8381-3305-8

Imprint (only for USA, GB)
Bibliographic information published by the Deutsche Nationalbibliothek: The Deutsche Nationalbibliothek lists this publication in the Deutsche Nationalbibliografie; detailed bibliographic data are available in the Internet at http://dnb.d-nb.de.
Any brand names and product names mentioned in this book are subject to trademark, brand or patent protection and are trademarks or registered trademarks of their respective holders. The use of brand names, product names, common names, trade names, product descriptions etc. even without a particular marking in this works is in no way to be construed to mean that such names may be regarded as unrestricted in respect of trademark and brand protection legislation and could thus be used by anyone.

Cover image: www.ingimage.com

Publisher: Südwestdeutscher Verlag für Hochschulschriften GmbH & Co. KG
Heinrich-Böcking-Str. 6-8, 66121 Saarbrücken, Germany
Phone +49 681 37 20 271-1, Fax +49 681 37 20 271-0
Email: info@svh-verlag.de

Printed in the U.S.A.
Printed in the U.K. by (see last page)
ISBN: 978-3-8381-3305-8

Acknowledgements

This work was supported by the "Medical-Scientific Fund of the Mayor of Vienna" (Project Number 08012).

Special thanks go to my PhD supervisors, Prof. Dr. Bernd Jilma and Prof. Dr. Robert Mader; Medical University of Vienna.

Moreover, I am grateful to the entire study team for the support in conducting the trial.

TABLE OF CONTENTS

1 INTRODUCTION

1.1 RHEUMATOID ARTHRITIS

1.1.1   PREVALENCE

Affecting approximately 1% of the adult world population, rheumatoid arthritis (RA) is the most common inflammatory joint disease. Women have a two-fold higher risk of developing the disease than men. The onset of disease typically occurs between the third and fifth decade of life [1] and is characterized by autoimmune destruction of multiple joints causing symptoms like pain, swelling, morning stiffness and loss of mobility [2]. Primarily, inflammation affects small single diarthrodial joints on hands and feet, but the disease progresses in a very rapid way and shortly destroys multiple joints – therefore called "polyarthritis".

As a chronic and systemic disease, rheumatoid arthritis targets synovial joints and is often accompanied by extra-articular manifestations. So the cardiovascular system and multiple other organ systems may be affected. Because of the work-disability of patients, the disease has economic consequences with related costs having a great impact on the health budget [3].

1.1.2   PATHOGENESIS

Although the causes of rheumatoid arthritis are not fully understood, several cell types including B-cells, T-cells, chondrocytes and osteoclasts are involved in the pathogenesis of the disease [4]. Further, synovial fibroblasts are discussed to play a central role through mediation of pathways of joint destruction, even in disease initiation.

After activation, synovial fibroblasts produce cytokines and chemokines in the rheumatoid synovium, which interact with inflammatory and endothelial cells. As a consequence, T-cells, macrophages and neutrophils are recruited, attracting more and more inflammatory cells [5]. The pannus, a granulation tissue formed by inflammation cells, invades and destroys local articular structures by the expression of degradative enzymes including metalloproteinases, serine proteases and aggrecanases [6] (pathway shown in figure 1).

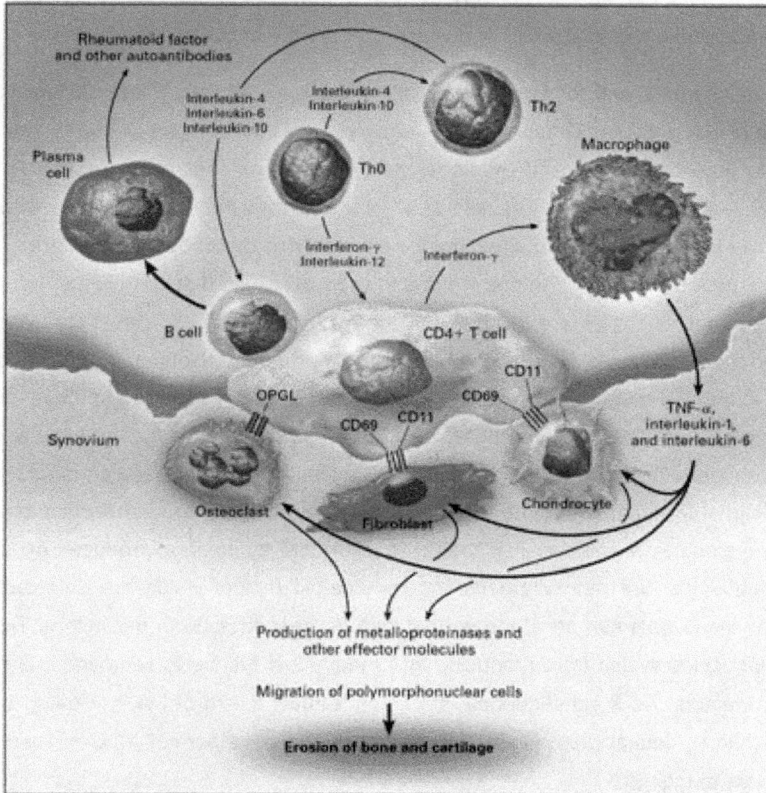

Figure 1: Cytokine Signaling Pathways Involved in Inflammatory Arthritis (Choy, NEJM 2001): The major cell types and cytokine pathways believed to be involved in joint destruction mediated by TNF-α and interleukin-1 are shown. Th2 denotes type 2 helper T cell, Th0 precursor of type 1 and type 2 helper T cells, and OPGL osteoprotegerin ligand

Therefore, joint damage occurs very early in rheumatoid arthritis with patients showing radiographic changes within two years after the onset of disease [7].

Another characteristic for the disease is the presence of rheumatoid factors in the serum of RA patients. These factors – observed for the first time in 1939 - are present in 80% of patients and predict a more aggressive course of disease. Almost twenty years later in 1957, Franklin et al. characterized these factors as antibodies that bind to the Fc portion of immunglobulins, showing that rheumatoid arthritis is an autoimmune disease [6]. Further, Neumann et al. observed that complement proteins and rheumatoid factors are produced in the synovium itself [8]. The Cy2-Cy3 interface in the Fc region of immunoglobulins is an important antigenic target for rheumatoid factors. An enzyme modification of self antigen is supposed to contribute to the pathogenesis of rheumatoid arthritis. In case of RA, rheumatoid factors have access to an epitope characterized by an absent galactose within the Fc region of IgG. With monoclonal rheumatoid factors binding better to agalactosyl IgG, antibodies against these molecules are raised in RA. Poly-reactive IgM antibodies, produced by CD5+ B-lymphocytes, are naturally occurring rheumatoid factors which are detectable in healthy individuals as part of the normal immune response. With the help of T-cells, B-lymphocytes switch from producing IgM rheumatoid factors to secreting IgG rheumatoid factors. As a consequence, the immune mechanism of RA is initiated by an HLA (human leukocyte antigen)-DR-restricted and T-helper-cell (CD4+)-mediated response to IgG [9].

Certain HLA polymorphisms are associated with RA, indicating a strong genetic influence. The HLA-DR gene resides in the major histocompatibility complex (MHC). The main function of HLA class II molecules is to present antigenic peptides to CD4+ T-cells, which might cause RA and influence the severity of disease [10]. Because synovitis is dependent on T-cells, synovial inflammation is influenced by HLA polymorphisms [11]. The shared epitope in the third hypervariable region of the DRB1 molecule is associated with the disease. This sequence is found on several DR4 positive alleles (i.e. *0401, *0404, *0405) as well as in some non-DR4 alleles (i.e. *0101, *1001) [12].

10

The influence of DRB1 genotype on RA phenotype could be related to the production of cytokines involved in cartilage erosions [13].

The role of cytokines in the pathogenesis of rheumatoid arthritis shall be illustrated in more detail. Firestein and colleagues observed that in RA synovium and synovial fluid T-cell cytokines such as Interleukin (IL)-2 and IFN (Interferon)-γ accumulated in lower concentrations than macrophage and fibroblast products such as IL-1, IL-6, IL-15, IL-18, TNF (Tumor Necrosis Factor) and GM-CSF (Granulocyte Macrophage – Colony Stimulating Factor) [14]. By inducing cartilage degradation, IL-1 and TNF promote inflammatory response and are therefore pro-inflammatory cytokines. In contrast, anti-inflammatory cytokines such as IL-4 or IL-10 neutralize the effect of pro-inflammatory molecules [15]. Therefore, the interaction of pro- and anti-inflammatory cytokines is an important approach for new therapeutic interventions in rheumatoid arthritis.

1.1.3   THERAPY OF RHEUMATOID ARTHRITIS

Disease-Modifying Antirheumatic Drugs (DMARDs), including methotrexate (MTX), leflunomide, hydroxychloroquine, D-penicillamine and gold salts as examples, slow the natural course of the disease by reduction of joint damage including pain and re-tarding loss of fuction. Therefore, in combination with Non-Steroidal Anti-Rheumatic Drugs (NSARs) and corticosteroids, DMARDs are the basis of RA therapy and are adequate in many patients.

However, DMARDs are discontinued because of inefficacy in 25% of patients or because of adverse events in 20% of patients [16, 17].

As a consequence, the development and application of new therapies for rheumatoid arthritis is of particular interest. Interacting with the inflammatory network, anti-TNF-α agents, IL-1 receptor antagonists, B-cell depletion and targeted cytokine immuno-therapies make a new approach in the therapy of rheumatoid arthritis [7].

Nevertheless, due to its positive benefit-risk ratio methotrexate remains the first-line drug in the treatment of rheumatoid arthritis not responsive to NSARs alone and is still in focus of research.

1.2 THE USE OF METHOTREXATE IN RHEUMATOID ARTHRITIS

Methotrexate, a folate antagonist, was originally developed for the treatment of cancer in the early 1950s. In 1948, the pediatric pathologist Sydney Farber observed that folic acid stimulated leukemic cell growth. In clinical practice, he demonstrated that the antimetabolite aminopterin – a chemical analogue of folic acid interfering with folate metabolism - produced temporary remissions in 25% of patients with acute lymphoblastic leukemia (ALL). Because of its toxic effects - in example nausea, vomiting, renal failure and abortions in pregnant woman - aminopterin was supplanted by the less toxic and equipotent methotrexate, which has become a cornerstone in the treatment of leukemia and other malignancies [18, 19]. In a way of targeted therapy, the inhibition of dihydrofolate reductase (DHFR) - an enzyme which participates in the tetrahydrofolate synthesis - leads to an impaired synthesis of DNA, RNA, thymidylates and proteins. Because of the fact that MTX acts during the S-phase of the cell cycle, rapidly dividing cells such as malignant cells are affected to a greater extent than normal dividing cells. This explains the relatively low incidence of toxicity and side effects. In case of rheumatoid arthritis, this cytotoxic effect is related to inflammatory cells. It was found, that mature T-lymphocytes are susceptible to T-cell-receptor mediated apoptosis during the S-phase of the cell cycle [19]. In this process, DNA synthesis is much more affected in duodenal mucosal cells than in bone marrow cells, explaining the gastrointestinal side effects of methotrexate [20].

Since its common use in rheumatology started after the publication of four controlled studies in 1985 [21], methotrexate is a mainstay in the therapy of rheumatoid arthritis and the most widely used DMARD worldwide – the "anchor drug" in rheumatoid arthritis [22].

In rheumatology, the drug is administered weekly in doses between 5 and 25 mg per week by oral or parenteral route.

In general, MTX is well tolerated and because of its positive benefit-risk ratio first-line therapy in rheumatoid arthritis. An important benefit is the possibility to adapt doses individually depending on the patient's disease status [23].

If introduced early in the course of disease, methotrexate is able to prevent or slow down disease progression with patients having significantly fewer new erosions and higher levels of radiographic stabilization than patients treated with other DMARDs [24]. In a study conducted by Weinblatt and colleagues, erosions were improved or unchanged in 8 of 14 patients who took MTX over 3 years [25].

Although in general MTX is very effective, the major drawback is the large inter-patient variability in clinical response. Defined by the "American College of Rheumatology (ACR)-20-criteria", clinical response is estimated to be between 46 and 65% [26, 27]. Because the drug is eliminated from plasma within 24 hours [28], serum levels are not suitable for drug monitoring, since methotrexate is efficacious for one week due to intracellular storage. Plasma concentrations just allow making a statement about a single compartment and not about the actual storage location. Therefore, serum concentrations are unreliable to measure clinical response. In contrast, the circulating intracellular levels of MTX polyglutamates (MTXPG) in erythrocytes are supposed to correlate with clinical efficacy [29]. For this reason, these metabolites may serve as potential markers for clinical response.

Further, toxicity is potentially limiting the use of MTX. It is estimated, that 10 to 30% of patients with rheumatoid arthritis withdraw from methotrexate-based therapy due to toxic effects [30]. To avoid severe side effects such as hematologic disorders and impaired renal and hepatic function, toxicity monitoring is performed routinely with blood counts and liver function tests. This protective measure results in the highest monitoring costs among the non-biologic DMARDs, although methotrexate itself is inexpensive [31].

All these facts require an improvement in the treatment with MTX to achieve a much more efficient and safe therapy for patients with rheumatoid arthritis.

1.2.1 PHARMACOLOGY

1.2.1.1 Chemical structure

Methotrexate (2,4-diamino-N^{10}-methylpteroylglutamic acid) is a weak bicarboxylic acid with the chemical IUPAC name (2S)-2-[[4-[(2,4-diaminopteridin-6-yl)methyl-methylamino]-benzoyl]amino]pentanedioic acid with the chemical formula $C_{20}H_{22}N_8O_5$. MTX is structurally related to folic acid with an amino-substitution instead of hydroxyl at position 4 and hydrogen substituted by a methyl-group at position 10.

The structure of folic acid (pteroylglutamic acid) consists of three connected elements:

- A pteridine ring system (composed of a pyrazine ring and a pyrimidine ring)

- Para-aminobenzoic acid

- A terminal glutamic acid residue

The chemical structures of methotrexate and folic acid are given in figure 2.

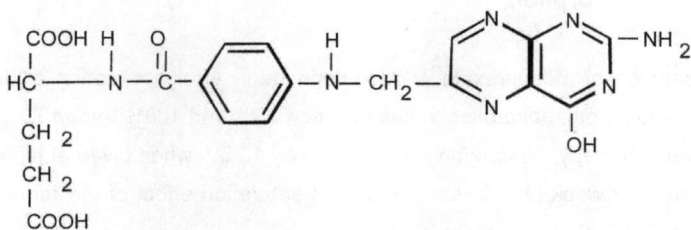

Folic Acid

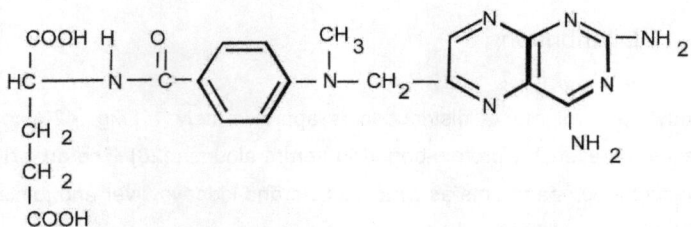

Methotrexate

Figure 2: Chemical structure of folic acid and methotrexate
(http://emedicine.medscape.com/article/200184-media, last checked 26/07/2010)

1.2.1.2   Absorption

Oral absorption of methotrexate is dose-dependent. After application of doses between 10 and 25 mg, absorption varies between 25% and 100% (mean 70%). During the course of therapy, absorption was reduced by 13.5% when given at higher doses than 17 mg per week [32], possibly due to a saturation effect of the reduced folate carrier (RFC) 1 [33].

1.2.1.3   Distribution

The steady-state volume of distribution is approximately 1 L/kg. 42% to 57% of methotrexate is reversibly protein-bound to serum albumin [28]. The drug distributes to extravascular compartments as synovial fluid and kidneys, liver and joints. Finally, a carrier-mediated active transport process takes up methotrexate into the cells [28].

1.2.1.4   Transport

Methotrexate is transported within the cell through the folate receptor (FR)-ß [34] and enters the cell via active transport by solute carrier family 19 member A1 (SLC19A1), also called reduced folate carrier. MTX is effluxed from the cell by members of the ATP-binding cassette (ABC) family of transporters. Multidrug resistance proteins (MRP) 1 and 3 represent components of the cellular efflux system for MTX. It was shown, that MRP3 is effective in transport of MTX and of folic acid, but that polyglutamation of MTX abolishes transport [35]. The circumstance that polyglutamates are retained within the cells to a higher extent than the main drug and folic acid, may indicate the importance of these metabolites as active products and explains the prolonged duration of intracellular storage.

1.2.1.5   Metabolism

Undergoing hepatic metabolism, approximately 10% of the major drug is converted to its main metabolite 7-hydroxy-methotrexate (7-OH-MTX), catalyzed by the enzyme aldehyde oxidase. 7-OH-MTX is over 90% bound to serum albumin. Intracellulary, both methotrexate and 7-OH-MTX are converted to polyglutamyl derivates by the enzyme folylpolyglutamate synthetase (FPGS). Polyglutamation can be reversed by the enzyme gamma-glutamyl hydrolase (GGH), which facilitates MTX efflux from the cell by catalyzing the removal of gamma-linked polyglutamates.

Polyglutamated MTX, which can have up to seven glutamic acid moieties (MTXPG2-7), has several important functions. It retains MTX within the cell [36], and inhibits DHFR (dihydrofolate reductase), an enzyme which reduces dihydrofolate (DHF) to tetrahydrofolate (THF). THF is the precursor of the biologically active folate cofactor 5-methyl THF, which is required for the generation of methionine from homocysteine and for the synthesis of polyamines [37]. Polyglutamated MTX also inhibits thymidylate synthase (TYMS), which converts deoxyuridylate to deoxythymidylate in the *de novo* pyrimidine biosynthetic pathway [38]. The enzyme N^5,N^{10}-methylenetetrahydrofolate reductase (MTHFR) in the folic acid pathway is not a direct target of MTX, but is influenced by the drug due to its effects on the intracellular folate pool. Because of these functions, the concentration of MTX polyglutamates in erythrocytes is supposed to correlate with therapeutic efficacy [39].

1.2.1.6   Elimination

The drug is excreted primarily by the kidneys, so 50% to 80% of the intact drug is renally eliminated through glomerular filtration [23]. After filtration, methotrexate is secreted and re-absorbed within the tubule. The mean elimination half-life is 5 to 8 hours, the mean renal clearance was observed to be between 4.8 and 7.8 L/h [28].

A small amount of MTX is excreted in the feces, probably via the bile (AHFS Drug Information).

As already mentioned, serum MTX is eliminated within 24 hours. In contrast, MTX polyglutamates present intracellular storage products which are retained up to one week in erythrocytes. Because MTX polyglutamates are supposed to be the active form of the main drug, their quantification seems suitable for drug monitoring to select patients responding to MTX-based therapy.

1.2.2   MODE OF ACTION

Although several theories have been proposed, detailed mechanisms of action in rheumatoid arthritis remain unclear.

As potential pharmacological mechanisms of action, the inhibition of purine and pyrimidine synthesis, the suppression of transmethylation reactions with accumulation of polyamines, the reduction of antigen-dependent T-cell proliferation and an adenosine-mediated suppression of inflammation come into consideration [33].

As a folate analogue, MTX inhibits dihydrofolate reductase. Consequently, less reduced folate (THF) is available for the *de novo* synthesis of purine and pyrimidine, which are important precursors of DNA and RNA.

Of particular interest for the indication of rheumatoid arthritis is that MTX acts as an anti-inflammatory agent in addition to its anti-proliferative effects.

In part, anti-inflammatory effects of MTX are mediated by extracellular adenosine increase through MTXPGs affinity for the enzyme AICAR (5-aminoimidazole-4-carboxamide ribonucleotide) transformylase. The AICAR enzyme system is a folate cofactor and plays a central role in the purine metabolism, leading to enhanced release of adenosine into the blood. The increase of AICAR inhibits two enzymes - AMP (adenosine monophosphate) deaminase and adenosine deaminase - and therefore the degradation of adenosine-5′-phosphate and adenosine [40-42].

Extracellular adenosine can bind to several transmembrane-spanning adenosine surface receptor types [43]. Methotrexate was found to induce extracellular adenosine acting predominantly through A2a receptors, which are coupled to $G\alpha_S$. Adenosine binding on A2 receptors inhibits lymphocyte proliferation and production of TNF, IL-8 and IL-12. Through the action on A3 receptors, adenosine leads to an inhibition of TNF, IL-12 and IFN-γ [44]. In contrast, the secretion of monocytic cytokines as IL-6 and IL-10 is hardly affected by methotrexate [45].

In addition, adenosine inhibits neutrophil adherence to endothelial cells and consequently neutrophil chemotaxis to inflammatory sites [46], altogether resulting in an anti-inflammatory action.

Supporting this theory, the results of Montesinos and co-workers provide strong evidence that adenosine mediates the anti-inflammatory effects of methotrexate in RA. They showed that the administration of the nonselective adenosine receptor antagonists theophylline and caffeine reversed anti-inflammatory effects of methotrexate in rats. Consequently, abstinence from caffeine may enhance the therapeutic effects of methotrexate in the treatment of rheumatoid arthritis [47]. It was even found, that coffee could reverse some benefits of methotrexate [48].

1.2.3   TOXICITY AND SIDE EFFECTS

Some adverse events of methotrexate seem to be related to its effect on purine and pyrimidine biosynthesis [33]. Therefore, folate supplementation was shown to reduce MTX toxicity, but was also discussed to reduce MTX efficacy. However, in several studies folate supplementation did not interfere with MTX efficacy [49]. On the other hand, improvement in MTX tolerability may be due to a relative dose reduction of MTX in patients taking folate supplementation [23]. However, the use of folate reduces plasma homocysteine levels, but not necessarily the risk for coronary artery disease due to hyperhomocysteinemia [50, 51].

Because methotrexate and folic acid compete for the same transporter for absorption and cellular uptake [52], patients are advised to supplement 5 mg folic acid 24 to 48 hours after MTX administration [53].

In general, 60-85% of patients report adverse events and 10-30% discontinue MTX due to toxicity [23]. Although clinically relevant side effects are rare, hepatotoxicity and gastrointestinal adverse events are the main reason for MTX withdrawal [54]. Further side effects are affecting the CNS (headache, dizziness), the hematopoietic system and the respiratory tract. Additionally, stomatitis, alopecia and bone marrow suppression are commonly encountered.

To detect toxicities and side effects in a timely manner, the American College of Rheumatology recommends to monitor liver function (alanine aminotransferase, aspartate aminotransferase, alkaline phosphatase, albumin and bilirubin) as well as hematologic values every 4 to 8 weeks during methotrexate therapy. In addition, liver blood tests, hepatitis B and C serologic studies and other standard tests including complete blood cell count and serum creatinine tests should be performed prior to starting treatment with MTX [55].

1.2.4 RESISTANCE

Resistance to methotrexate is a phenomenon characterized by gradual reduction in drug efficacy. These mechanisms are based on loss of the ability to block the release of pro-inflammatory cytokines and on limited anti-proliferative effects [17].

Morgan and colleagues showed, that multidrug resistance to DMARDs affects 5% of patients [56], therefore presenting an uncommon but important problem.

In cancer as well as in rheumatoid arthritis, several mechanisms of cellular resistance to methotrexate are discussed. The underlying molecular cause for loss of efficacy of anti-rheumatic drugs is not fully understood, but might be mediated by mechanisms shared with anticancer drugs [17].

In experimental tumors was shown, both *in vitro* and *in vivo*, that drug transport via RFC or FR can be impaired through decreased protein levels, altered kinetics or a lower affinity of the receptor for methotrexate than for folic acid. Further, drug efflux via ABC subfamily transporters ABCC1-ABCC5 and ABCG2 can be increased. In addition, an impaired metabolism of methotrexate may contribute to cellular resistance. On the one hand, activity of GGH (which degrades polyglutamate residues) and concentrations of 7-hydroxymethotrexate may be elevated. On the other hand, expression of the enzyme FPGS might be decreased with the consequence of an impaired polyglutamation of methotrexate. Moreover, altered target enzymes possibly lead to drug resistance, for example through increased DHFR activity or expression [17, 57, 58].

Increased ABCB1 expression was also discussed to play a role in resistance to methotrexate [59]. But due to the fact that this transporter prefers neutral or cationic compounds, the relation to MTX as an anionic drug is questionable [60].

Against all expectations, the observation of Stranzl and colleagues showed a negative correlation of mRNA levels of FPGS and response to methotrexate in patients with rheumatoid arthritis [61]. Consequently, these results indicate that FPGS is involved in the resistance to methotrexate in rheumatoid arthritis patients.

In addition to the mentioned mechanisms, several common polymorphisms coding for folate or methotrexate transporters were defined and correlate with response to methotrexate. The genotypes 80AA in the RFC region, 347GG in the AICAR transformylase region and 1298CC and 677CC in the MTHFR region may serve as examples for a greater clinical improvement [62, 63].

The understanding of these mechanisms is required to develop potent strategies to overcome MTX resistance. For the therapy of cancer, second-generation folate antagonists were designed, which are more efficiently taken up by RFC and better substrates for FPGS. In rheumatology, the combination with other DMARDs and alternating drugs is an appropriate approach to prevent resistance [17, 57].

1.2.5 PHARMACOGENOMICS AND PHARMACOGENETICS OF METHOTREXATE

Pharmacogenomics and pharmacogenetics are new fields to optimize drug therapy by improving safety and reducing adverse events.

Pharmacogenetics is the science of genetic variations involved in drug metabolism and is a tool to predict drug effectiveness and drug-induced adverse events.

The most common form of genetic variations is the single nucleotide polymorphism (SNP). In this case, a single nucleotide base is altered or deleted, or an additional nucleotide base is inserted.

Due to its metabolism and mechanism of action, some potential genes are reported to be associated with response to or toxicity of MTX. A number of enzymes mediating MTX metabolism (DHFR, TYMS, FPGS, GGH, AICAR, ATIC, MTHFR) are of particular interest. The C677T polymorphism in the MTHFR region for example is associated with enhanced bone-marrow toxicity. Further, polymorphisms affecting the transporter RFC influence the efficacy of MTX [64].

Because the main focus of this work is on gene expression analysis of cytokines and involved enzymes in polyglutamation (FPGS, GGH), SNPs are not described in detail at this point.

Gene expression works at the transcriptional level and may be investigated using several techniques. Among them, one is real-time reverse transcriptase PCR (polymerase chain reaction), which for instance allows looking for the modulation of immunoregulatory cytokines by methotrexate during the course of treatment. As a result, insight into therapeutic targets of methotrexate is provided.

It was previously shown, that MTX increases IL-4 and IL-10 gene expression in peripheral blood mononuclear cells (PBMC) in rheumatoid arthritis patients. IL-2 and IFN-γ are decreased while using methotrexate, explaining its immunoregulatory action in rheumatoid arthritis [65]. To gain new knowledge about the anti-inflammtory effect of methotrexate, further genes of the cytokine network need to be studied.

1.3 OPEN QUESTIONS

As already mentioned, methotrexate is a cornerstone in the therapy of rheumatoid arthritis. Although the drug is very effective, the large inter-patient variability regarding efficacy and the frequency of adverse events are major drawbacks.

Despite its use in rheumatoid arthritis over several decades, some questions concerning clinical practice remained open.

First of all, there is a controversial discussion if methotrexate polyglutamates play an essential role in drug response and if their concentration may serve as potential markers for the efficacy of methotrexate. In contrast to Dervieux and colleagues, who stated that the concentrations of erythrocyte polyglutamates with three or more glutamic residues are associated with therapeutic response [39], Stamp et al. showed that polyglutamate concentrations do not correlate with disease activity [66]. However, all these studies did not include the measurement of erythrocyte blank values before starting MTX. Therefore, important information on polyglutamation per se is unavailable, because it is not clarified if polyglutamates may occur as natural products in erythrocytes. This lack of information makes it difficult to understand the formation of these metabolites.

Secondly, it is not well established if methotrexate should be started using conventional doses up to 15 mg per week or immediately at higher doses.

In a prospective, non-blinded trial Schnabel and co-workers enrolled 185 patients with rheumatoid arthritis receiving either an initial dose of 15 mg or 25 mg methotrexate per week. As a result, gastrointestinal side effects were significantly more common in patients receiving 25 mg methotrexate (P<0.05). Further, liver enzymes were elevated to a higher extent than in the 15 mg group [67].

Another trial showed that increasing doses up to 45 mg/week administered parenterally did not improve disease control [68]. The results may indicate that higher doses entail a higher risk for adverse events without a gain in efficacy.

In contrast, Visser and Van der Heijde stated in their systematic review, that higher starting doses using 25 mg MTX per week are associated with higher efficacy, but also with higher toxicity compared to lower doses or slow escalation [69]. Therefore, this topic remains controversial.

Finally, there are ongoing discussions about differences in efficacy of methotrexate after subcutaneous administration versus oral dosing.

The bioavailability of methotrexate is reduced by up to 40% when administered orally. At higher doses of 17 mg per week, Hamilton and group observed a significant increase in AUC when MTX was given i.m. compared to the oral route [32]. As a consequence, switching from oral to parenteral administration is recommended to improve bioavailability.

It is also inconsistent if the parenteral administration diminishes adverse events. In one study, more withdrawal due to toxicity was observed [70]. In contrast, observational data indicate that gastrointestinal side effects are reduced when using subcutaneous administration [71].

To make a contribution to answer the mentioned questions, the study presented in the thesis project at hand was designed.

The aims of the project were to investigate the correlation of methotrexate polyglutamate concentrations with clinical response and to compare the efficacy of a conventional starting dose with a higher starting dose.

In addition, real time PCR was performed to evaluate the impact of methotrexate-based therapy on the gene expression of selected pro-inflammatory cytokines such as TNF, IL-6, IL-12A, IL-17A and IL-18 and enzymes being involved in drug metabolism (FPGS, GGH) in patients with rheumatoid arthritis.

2 CLINICAL PART

2.1 BACKGROUND OF THE STUDY

Methotrexate is the most-widely used DMARD in the treatment of rheumatoid arthritis. Despite its positive benefit-risk ratio, some questions - presented in detail in the introduction - remain open.

Primarily, these questions are related to the mode of action of MTX and the impact of methotrexate polyglutamates on clinical response in rheumatoid arthritis.

Therefore, the primary aims were to study the pharmacokinetics of MTX as well as MTX polyglutamates and to investigate if erythrocyte levels of MTX polyglutamates are associated with clinical response in rheumatoid arthritis.

The second purpose of the trial was to compare efficacy and safety of a standard dose versus a higher starting dose. The idea was that a higher starting dose of 25 mg MTX per week may accelerate clinical response to a higher extent than a standard dose of 15 mg per week in MTX-naïve patients. Moreover, the incidence of side effects should be compared by the use of two different dosing schemata.

In addition, the influence of MTX-based therapy on the gene expression of key cytokines involved in the pathogenesis of rheumatoid arthritis (TNF, IL-6, IL-12A, IL-17A and IL-18) as well as of FPGS and GGH should be investigated using real-time PCR technique.

2.2 MATERIALS AND METHODS

2.2.1 *USED TOOLS FOR DIAGNOSIS OF RHEUMATOID ARTHRITIS*

2.2.1.1 American College of Rheumatology Criteria

In 1987, the *American College of Rheumatology* has defined the following *criteria for classification* of rheumatoid arthritis [72]:

- Morning stiffness (lasting at least for 1 hour before maximal improvement)

- Arthritis of three or more joint areas

- Arthritis of hand joints

- Symmetric arthritis

- Rheumatoid nodules

- Serum rheumatoid factor positivity

- Radiographic changes

For classification purposes, four of these seven points have to be fulfilled.

2.2.1.2 Disease Activity Score in 28 joints (DAS-28)

The *DAS-28* is a measure of disease activity of rheumatoid arthritis and is the golden standard in clinical practice and research. In calculation, the following parameters are included:

- Number of tender joints (TEN)

- Number of swollen joints (SW)

- Erythrocyte sedimentation rate (ESR)

- Patient assessment of disease activity (VAS, mm)

The DAS-28 is calculated using the following formula:

$$0.56 \times \sqrt{TEN28} + 0.28 \times \sqrt{SW28} + 0.70 \times ln(ESR) + 0.014 \times (VAS) = DAS\text{-}28$$

Table 1 shows the evaluation of current DAS-28 and how to interpret the difference to initial values. The index allows classifying the activity and severity of disease and presents an appropriate tool to monitor the efficacy of DMARD-based therapy. Therapy with DMARDs should be started in patients with an active disease (DAS-28 $\geq$ 3.2) as soon as possible after making the diagnosis. The primary aim of therapy is to achieve remission in rheumatoid arthritis, defined as DAS-28 $\leq$ 2.6 (http://www.das-score.nl, last checked 30/07/2010). Because of the fact that this index is just a guide for monitoring the activity of disease, therapeutic decisions should not be made without considering subjective parameters of patients such as pain and restrictions in daily life.

Current DAS-28		Difference to initial value		
		> 1.2	> 0.6 ≤ 1.2	≤ 0.6
≤ 3.2	Inactive	Good Improvement	Moderate Improvement	No Improvement
> 3.2 ≤ 5.1	Moderate	Moderate Improvement	Moderate Improvement	No Improvement
> 5.1	Very Active	Moderate Improvement	No Improvement	No Improvement

Table 1: Evaluation of DAS-28

2.2.1.3   Health Assessment Questionnaire (HAQ)

The HAQ-Score, developed in 1980 at Stanford University, is a patient reported outcome to assess physical, social and emotional disabilities. The value of HAQ ranges from 0 to 3. Zero means no disabilities in daily life; a value of three reflects the highest possible handicap for patients [73].

2.2.2   STRUCTURE OF THE CLINICAL TRIAL

A randomized, double-blinded, controlled clinical trial phase 4 was performed in accordance with Good Clinical Practice (GCP) guidelines and ethical principles that have their origin in the Declaration of Helsinki.

After submission of the protocol to the ethics committee ("Ethikkommission der Stadt Wien") and obtaining approval in written, patient recruitment was started.

MTX-naïve patients who fulfilled the American College of Rheumatology criteria for rheumatoid arthritis were enrolled at the Department of Rheumatology at the Kaiser-Franz-Josef Hospital (SMZ Sued) in Vienna.

After informed consent, patients were screened and clinical status was assessed by the number of joint counts (DAS-28), HAQ-Score and laboratory parameters.

Because of the possibility of methotrexate-related pulmonary complications, the screening further involved a chest-x-ray to exclude pulmonary diseases.

Patients who fulfilled any of the following criteria had to be excluded from study participation:

- Previous use of MTX

- Persons younger than 18 years

- DAS-28 ≤ 3.2 (inactive rheumatoid arthritis)

- Pulmonary diseases

- Infectious diseases (HIV, hepatitis B and C)

- Gestation and lactation

- Contraindications for MTX according to product information

To compare the clinical response and efficacy of a standard and a higher starting dose, patients were randomly assigned to two different dosing schemata.

The first schema (standard dose) planned a starting dose of 15 mg MTX per week, administered orally. Afterwards, the dose was escalated every two weeks until a weekly dose of 25 mg was achieved at week 5.

The second schema (high dose) required to start immediately with 25 mg MTX per week, administered orally.

At week 5, all patients received a subcutaneous dose of 25 mg MTX to get a 100%-reference level for bioavailability. From week 6 to the end of the clinical trial at week 16, the oral dose of 25 mg per week was maintained.

Blinding was ensured through encapsulation of MTX.

Scheduled visits to collect blood for laboratory testing (complete blood counts) and pharmacokinetics were arranged at week 1, week 5, week 10 and at the end of study at week 16.

Among blood collections, disease status was evaluated in detail at the beginning and the end of trial, including assessment of the DAS-28 and HAQ-Score.

To prevent interactions with food and other drugs, patients were instructed to take MTX in a fasting state. Further, concomitant medication was recorded in detail.

For pharmacokinetic analysis, blood collections had to be carried out before and after drug administration at defined times, presented in table 2.

Week	Pre-value	1.5 hours	4 hours	48 hours	96 hours	168 hours
1	✓	✓	✓	✓	✓	✓
5	✓	✓	✓	✓	✓	✓
10	✓	✓	✓	✓	✓	✓
16	✓					

Table 2: Defined times for blood collections

The primary outcome parameter for evaluation was the DAS-28; secondary outcome parameters were the HAQ-Score, CRP, ESR, VAS pain and VAS fatigue.

For a better understanding of the study procedures, a flow chart is given in figure 3.

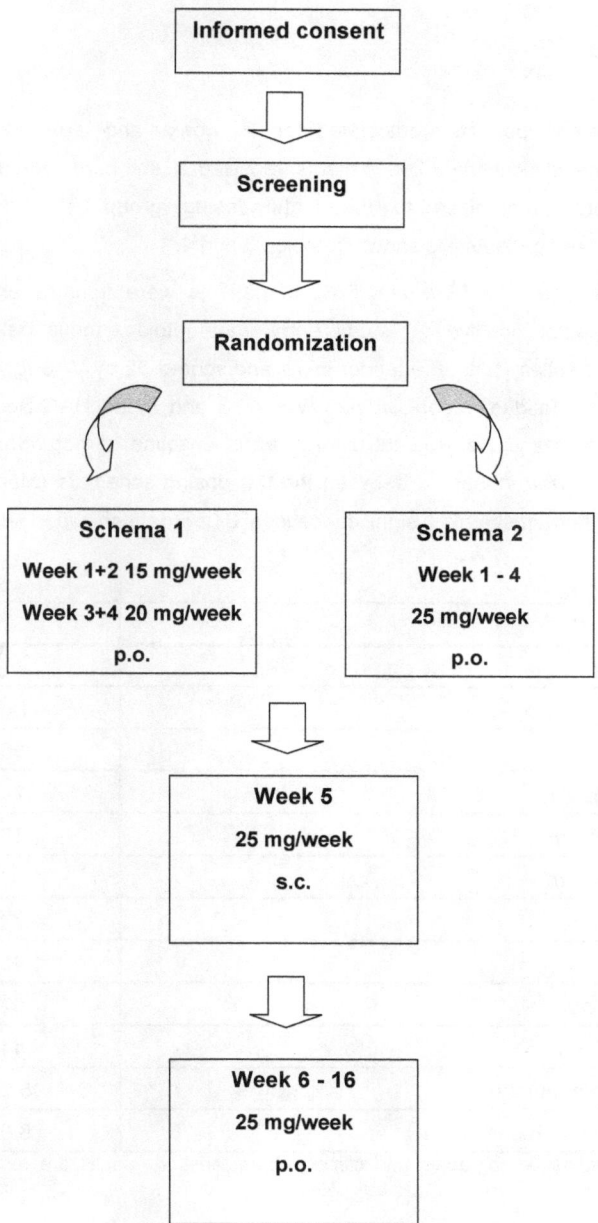

Figure 3: Flow Chart Study Procedures

2.3 RESULTS

Overall, nineteen patients participated for 16 weeks and therefore successfully concluded the clinical trial. Ten patients received a standard starting dose; nine patients were randomized to the higher-dosing group. The main baseline characteristics of patients are shown in tables 3 and 4.

The average age was 56 years. 68% of patients were females and 42% were rheumatoid factor positive. At study entry, rheumatoid arthritis patients had on average 5.2 swollen joints, 8.9 tender joints and scored 52 by VAS for joint pain and 44 by VAS for fatigue. Mean DAS-28 was 4.73 and mean HAQ-Score was 1.45. Further, no statistically significant differences in baseline demographic and clinical characteristics were observed between the two dosing schemata (Mann-Whitney-U-test for independent samples, significance level 0.05) (data shown in table 4).

Characteristic	
Sex, % (F/M)	68/32
Smoker, %	10.50
Age, yr	56 (± 13)
Body weight, kg	74 (± 12)
Body height, cm	167 (± 6)
Body surface, m²	1.83 (± 0.13)
DAS-28	4.73 (± 1.02)
HAQ-Score	1.45 (± 0.85)
Pain (VAS, mm)	52 (± 22)
Fatigue (VAS, mm)	44 (± 32)
Swollen joints, number	5.2 (± 6.0)
Tender joints, number	8.9 (± 7.4)

Table 3: Baseline demographic and clinical characteristics: results are expressed as the mean (SD)

Characteristic	Standard dose	High dose	Significance
Demographic*			
Patients, n	10	9	0.874
Sex, % (F/M)	70/30	67/33	0.884
Smoker, %	10	11	0.941
Age, yr	51 (± 15)	62 (± 7)	0.053
Body weight, kg	72 (± 14)	77 (± 8)	0.329
Body height, cm	165 (± 6)	170 (± 5)	0.109
Body surface, m²	1.78 (± 0.14)	1.88 (± 0.11)	0.106
Clinical			
DAS-28	4.93 (± 0.97)	4.50 (± 1.08)	0.288
HAQ-Score	1.54 (± 0.96)	1.35 (± 0.75)	0.935
Pain (VAS, mm)	55 (± 26)	50 (± 18)	0.588
Fatigue (VAS, mm)	56 (± 33)	32 (± 28)	0.107
Morning stiffness, min	53 (± 56)	46 (± 34)	0.889
Rheumatoid factor pos., %	50	33	0.475
Anti-CCP pos., %	30	22	0.874
ESR, mm/h	29.20 (± 19.28)	24.78 (± 20.61)	0.347
CRP, mg/dl	11.79 (± 15.23)	11.07 (± 15.73)	0.369
Hemoglobin, g/dl	13.06 (± 1.48)	13.33 (± 1.11)	0.775
Leukocytes, /nl	7.99 (± 2.85)	7.64 (± 3.54)	0.624
Lymphocytes, %	29.00 (± 8.51)	26.42 (± 6.94)	0.568
ANC, /nl	4.62 (± 1.97)	4.69 (± 2.52)	0.568
Basophils, %	0.51 (± 0.27)	0.74 (± 0.22)	0.077
Eosinophils, %	3.16 (± 2.11)	4.64 (± 4.22)	0.367
Monocytes, %	8.17 (± 2.59)	8.62 (± 2.06)	0.514
Creatinine, mg/dl	0.82 (± 0.22)	0.91 (± 0.23)	0.369

Table 4: Two group comparison of baseline demographic and clinical characteristics (Mann-Whitney-U-test for independent samples, *Student´s t-test for independent samples, significance level 0.05): results are expressed as the mean (SD)

As presented in table 5a, at week 5 laboratory analysis of inflammation parameters did not indicate a significant benefit of a higher starting dose (Mann-Whitney-U-test for independent samples). In contrast, levels of basophils and eosinophils were higher compared to the standard-dosing group. It is remarkable, that no elevation of liver function enzymes and no decrease in renal function were observed in the "high-dosing group".

Between-group-comparison showed no significant differences in DAS-28 and HAQ-Score at the end of study at week 16 (Mann-Whitney-U-test for independent samples) (table 5b).

Characteristic	Standard dose	High dose	Significance
ESR, mm/h	19.60 (± 17.40)	19.56 (± 14.75)	0.806
CRP, mg/dl	3.92 (± 2.22)	5.14 (± 3.86)	0.902
Leukocytes, /nl	7.62 (± 3.44)	6.65 (± 3.03)	0.288
Lymphocytes, %	28.57 (± 6.26)	28.97 (± 5.51)	0.806
ANC, /nl	4.81 (± 2.98)	3.96 (± 2.11)	0.369
Basophils, %	0.36 (± 0.26)	0.68 (± 0.35)	0.014*
Eosinophils, %	2.77 (± 2.14)	4.24 (± 2.37)	0.037*
Monocytes, %	7.87 (± 1.96)	7.86 (± 1.36)	0.713
Creatinine, mg/dl	0.78 (± 0.17)	0.91 (± 0.25)	0.153
Alkaline Phosphatase, U/l	73.40 (± 21.05)	66.11 (± 15.50)	0.191
ASAT, U/l	23.20 (± 8.09)	24.67 (± 4.77)	0.325
ALAT, U/l	30.20 (± 22.98)	28.00 (± 8.90)	0.624

Table 5a: Two-group-comparison of laboratory parameters at week 5 (Mann-Whitney-U-test for independent samples, significance level 0.05): results are expressed as the mean (SD)

Characteristic	Standard dose	High dose	Significance
DAS-28	2.87 (± 0.93)	2.66 (± 0.11)	1.000
Improvement in DAS-28	2.07 (± 1.39)	1.84 (± 0.83)	0.935
HAQ-Score	0.60 (± 0.46)	0.64 (± 0.57)	0.934
Improvement in HAQ-Score	1.00 (± 0.83)	0.71 (± 0.35)	0.566

Table 5b: Two-group-comparison of DAS-28 and HAQ-Score at week 16 (Mann-Whitney-U-test for independent samples, significance level 0.05): results are expressed as the mean (SD)

At the end of study at week 16, measurement of laboratory and clinical parameters demonstrated that MTX was significantly effective in reducing DAS-28, HAQ-Score, PGA (Patient´s global assessment), EGA (Evaluator´s global assessment), VAS pain, VAS fatigue, the number of swollen and tender joints as well as the duration of morning stiffness and rheumatoid factor (Wilcoxon-test for paired samples, significance level 0.05). ESR was significantly reduced using Student´s t test (p=0.039, CI 95%), but not when using Wilcoxon-test for paired samples (p=0.070, significance level 0.05). Surprisingly, other inflammatory parameters such as the CRP just showed a trend towards a reduction by the use of methotrexate (data shown in table 6). This may be explained by the limited sample size of the study.

Characteristic	Pre-value	Week 16	Significance
Scores			
DAS-28	4.73 (± 1.02)	2.77 (± 0.99)	0.000*
HAQ-Score	1.45 (± 0.85)	0.62 (± 0.50)	0.000*
Subjective parameters			
Pain (VAS, mm)	52 (± 22)	27 (± 22)	0.002*
Fatigue (VAS, mm)	44 (± 32)	29 (± 23)	0.018*
PGA (VAS, mm)	50 (± 20)	27 (± 15)	0.001*
EGA (VAS, mm)	51 (± 20)	27 (± 17)	0.001*
Clinical parameters			
Morning stiffness, min	50 (± 46)	29 (± 61)	0.050*
Swollen joints, number	5.2 (± 6.0)	1.6 (± 3.0)	0.005*
Tender joints, number	8.9 (± 7.4)	2.3 (± 3.4)	0.006*
Laboratory parameters			
Rheumatoid factor, U/l	50.24 (± 81.36)	23.20 (± 28.80)	0.006*
Anti-CCP, U/l	91.86 (± 171.11)	77.15 (± 130.11)	0.500
ESR, mm/h	27.11 (± 19.49)	18.32 (± 15.90)	0.070
CRP, mg/dl	11.45 (± 15.04)	3.89 (± 4.18)	0.076
Hemoglobin, g/dl	13.19 (± 1.29)	13.43 (± 1.15)	0.777
Leukocytes, /nl	7.82 (± 3.11)	7.35 (± 2.61)	0.546
Lymphocytes, %	27.78 (± 7.70)	24.41 (± 7.02)	0.334
ANC, /nl	4.65 (± 2.18)	4.82 (± 2.30)	0.494
Basophils, %	0.62 (± 0.27)	0.58 (± 0.40)	0.575
Eosinophils, %	3.86 (± 3.28)	3.11 (± 2.44)	0.133
Monocytes, %	8.38 (± 2.30)	8.39 (± 1.84)	0.653

Table 6: Efficacy of MTX - Comparison of clinical parameters (pre-value and week 16) (Wilcoxon-test for paired samples, significance level 0.05): results are expressed as the mean (SD)

It was shown, that methotrexate was highly effective regarding scores and subjective parameters. As presented in figure 4, the DAS-28 was significantly reduced when comparing week 16 with pre-values (2.77 ± 0.99 versus 4.73 ± 1.02, p=0.000).

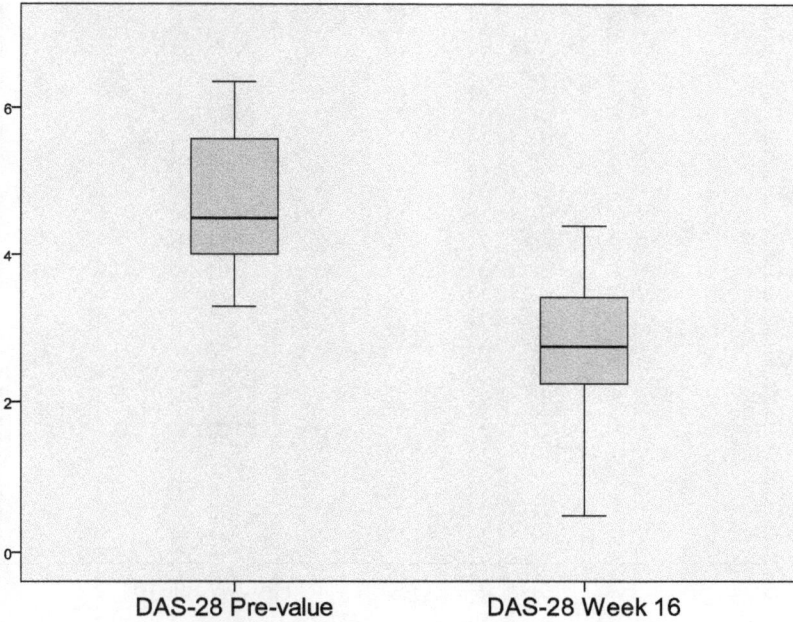

Figure 4: Box-and-Whisker plot DAS-28 (Comparison Pre-value and Week 16); values given as the median with 25th and 75th percentiles; min, max

Figure 5 illustrates changes in HAQ-Score. Comparing pre-values with week 16, the HAQ-Score was reduced from a mean of 1.45 (± 0.85) to a mean of 0.62 (± 0.50) (p≤0.001).

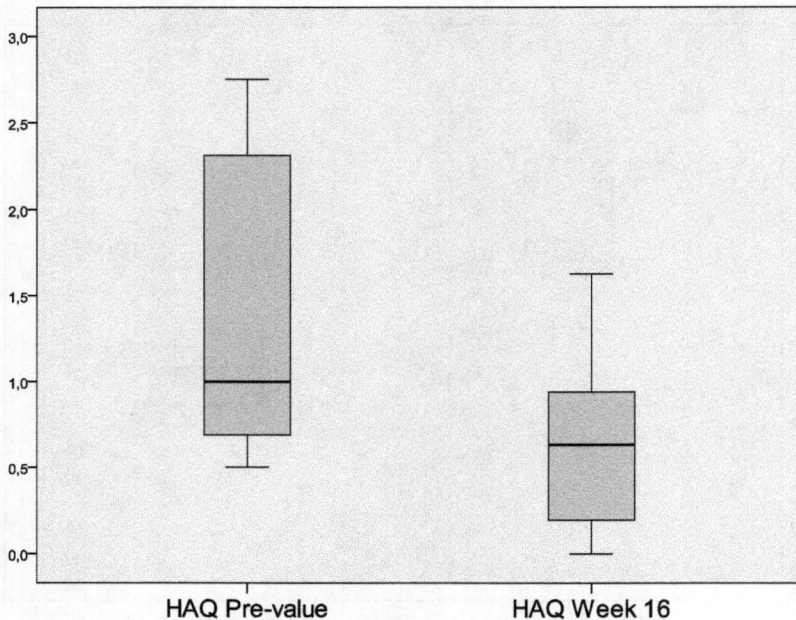

Figure 5: Box-and-Whisker plot HAQ-Score (Comparison Pre-value and Week 16); values given as the median with 25th and 75th percentiles; min, max

Representing other subjective parameters, patient´s global assessment (PGA) (p=0.001) as well as the evaluator´s global assessment (EGA) (p=0.001) were significantly reduced when using Wilcoxon-test for paired samples (figures 6 and 7).

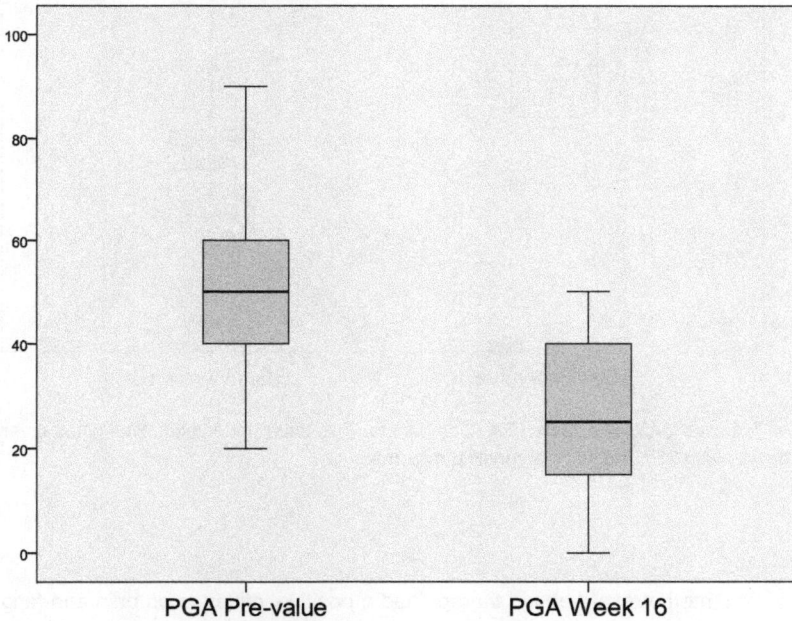

Figure 6: Box-and-Whisker plot PGA (Comparison Pre-value and Week 16), values given as the median with 25th and 75th percentiles; min, max

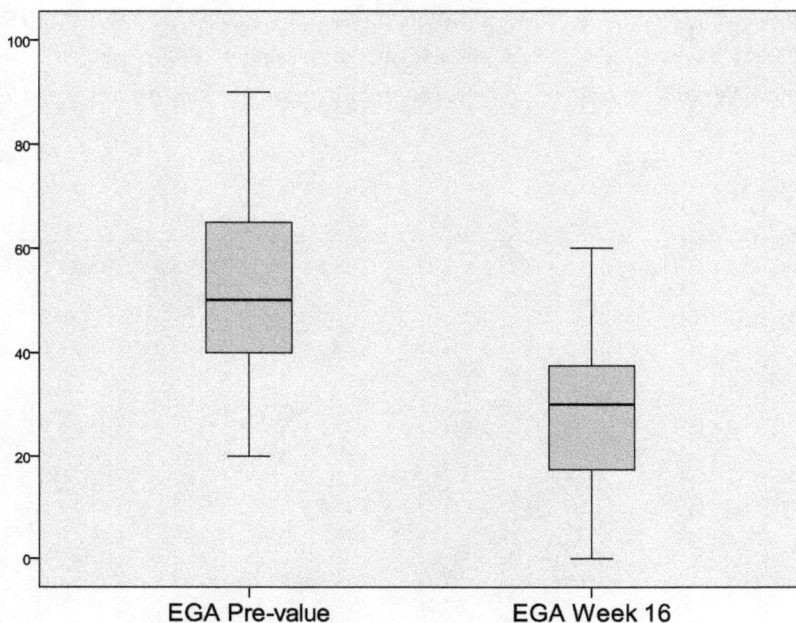

Figure 7: Box-and-Whisker plot EGA (Comparison Pre-value and Week 16), values given as the median with 25th and 75th percentiles; min, max

In addition, methotrexate-based therapy had a positive influence on pain and fatigue, which were quantified using Visual Analogue Scales (VAS).

VAS pain (mm) was reduced from a mean of 52 (± 22) to a mean of 27 (± 22) (p=0.002). Further, VAS fatigue (mm) was reduced from a mean of 44 (± 32) to a mean of 29 (± 23) (p=0.018) (Wilcoxon-test for paired samples). Results are shown in figures 8 and 9.

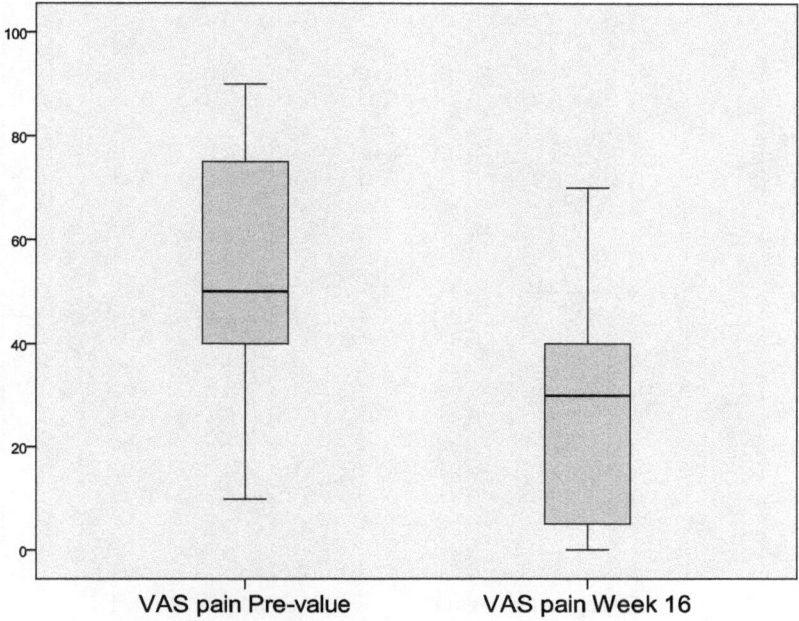

Figure 8: Box-and-Whisker plot VAS pain (Comparison Pre-value and Week 16), values given as the median with 25th and 75th percentiles; min, max

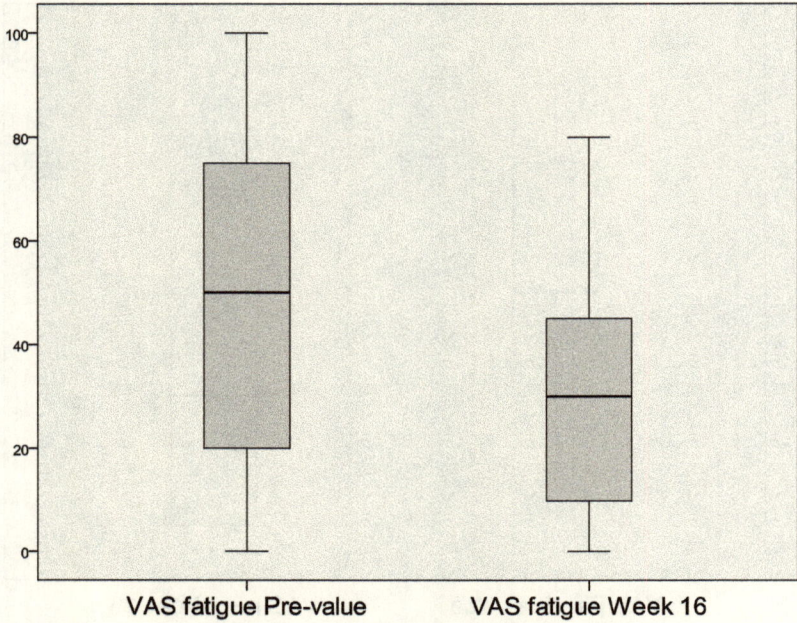

Figure 9: Box-and-Whisker plot VAS fatigue (Comparison Pre-value and Week 16), values given as the median with 25th and 75th percentiles; min, max

As illustrated in figure 10, ESR, an important inflammatory parameter, was significantly reduced using the Student´s t-test (p=0.039), but not when using the Wilcoxon-test for paired samples (p=0.070). This may be explained by the limited sample size of the study.

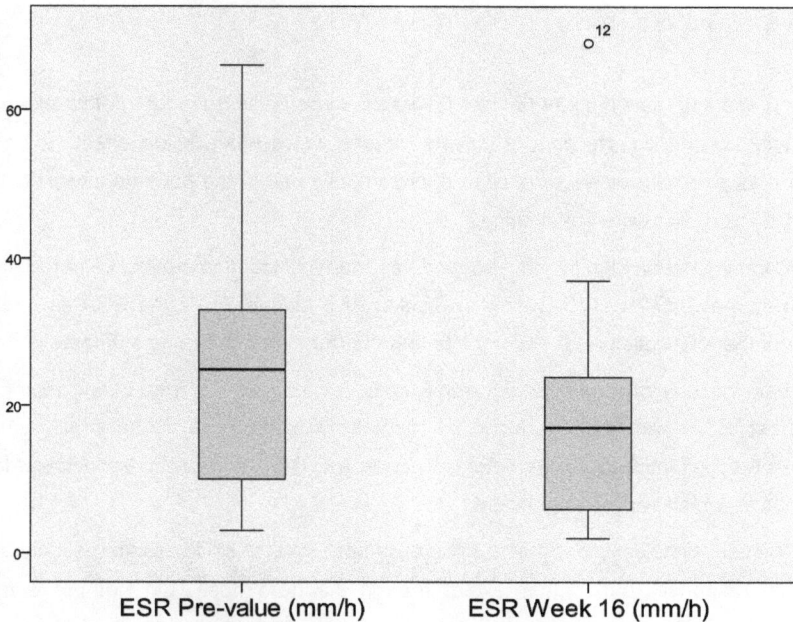

Figure 10: Box-and-Whisker plot ESR (mm/h) (Comparison Pre-value and Week 16), values given as the median with 25th and 75th percentiles; min, max

As a conclusion, methotrexate is highly effective in reducing subjective parameters as the DAS-28, HAQ-Score, VAS pain, VAS fatigue as well as PGA and EGA and the duration of morning stiffness. Further, the number of swollen (1.6 ± 3.0 versus 5.2 ± 6.0, p=0.005, Wilcoxon-test for paired samples) and tender joints (2.3 ± 3.4 versus 8.9 ± 7.4, p=0.006, Wilcoxon-test for paired samples) was influenced in a positive way by the use of MTX.

As a laboratory parameter, rheumatoid factor (U/l) was reduced from a mean of 50.24 (± 81.36) to a mean of 23.20 (± 28.80) (p=0.006, Wilcoxon-test for paired samples). Surprisingly, ESR was hardly influenced by the use of methotrexate. Due to the relatively small sample size, the trend towards a reduction in the CRP was not significant.

2.4 Discussion

The presented study confirms the favorable benefit-risk ratio of methotrexate in rheumatoid arthritis. No serious adverse events were noted. Side effects such as stomatitis and nausea were noted in approximately half of the patients after initiating MTX therapy, but were self-limiting.

MTX administration significantly reduced important clinical and subjective parameters such as the DAS-28, HAQ-Score, VAS pain, VAS fatigue, PGA and EGA as well as the number of swollen and tender joints and the duration of morning stiffness.

Further, the use of methotrexate significantly reduced serum rheumatoid factor. In contrast, ESR was hardly reduced by methotrexate. Because of the small sample size, other inflammatory parameters such as the CRP showed a trend towards a reduction, which was not significant.

The original consideration, that a higher starting dose of MTX possibly accelerates clinical response to a higher extent than a standard dose, did not prove true. Although no differences in side effects were observed, a starting dose of 15 mg per week should be recommended to prevent a potential impairment in liver and kidney function.

3 PHARMACOKINETICS

The next step of the project was to perform High pressure liquid chromatography (HPLC) analysis to investigate if erythrocyte polyglutamate levels and MTX plasma levels correlate with clinical response in rheumatoid arthritis.

3.1 INTRODUCTION

In rheumatoid arthritis, methotrexate is generally administered as a single weekly dose, given orally or subcutaneously. The usual dose is in the range of 15 to 20 mg per week. At these doses, the bioavailability varies individually but is in general approximately 70% after oral administration [74].

MTX is mainly absorbed in the proximal jejunum, whereas absorption may be reduced in case of intestinal pathology. Concomitant food intake does not influence absorption [75].

In the liver, a modest fraction of the MTX dose (~10%) is converted to the main metabolite 7-hydroxymethotrexate. Both MTX and 7-OH-MTX are primarily excreted in the urine with some biliary excretion. The half-life of MTX in the serum is in the range of 6 to 8 hours.

MTX is taken up by cells and polyglutamated up to seven glutamyl-residues (MTXPG 2-7). Because of the fact that these compounds are long-lived and active, the concentration of MTX polyglutamates is supposed to correlate with clinical efficacy [74]. In contrast, the major part of serum MTX is excreted by the kidneys within the first 12 hours after administration. Therefore, plasma MTX measurements alone are not very useful for drug monitoring.

However, the combination with measuring erythrocyte polyglutamates is an option to generate a complete pharmacokinetic profile of the drug, including the determination of long-lived storage products.

Hence, in this study two different HPLC approaches were used to get a detailed pharmacokinetic profile of the drug and its metabolites in different tissues – in plasma and erythrocytes.

As previously described by Yu and co-workers, *plasma MTX and 7-hydroxymethotrexate* were analyzed using an ion-pair chromatography in a column-switching system with an alkyl-diol silica (ADS) precolumn and post-column photochemical reaction [76, 77].

Using ADS, macromolecular compounds such as proteins were removed before HPLC analysis to prevent precipitation on column packing material and capillary obstruction. ADS columns consist of special reversed-phase sorbents to purify samples before being transferred onto the analytical column. At the outer surface of the spherical particles, hydrophilic and electroneutral diol groups are bound. Thereby, proteins can be directly flushed into the waste. The inner surface with hydrophobic alkyl chains is freely accessible for lower molecular analytes. There, the analytes are extracted and enriched. Finally, the purified sample is transferred onto the analytical column [78].

A two-column HPLC system for integrated sample preparation is illustrated in figure 11. The precolumn is connected via a 6-port switching valve to an analytical column. The 6-port valve, used for column switching, has no direct sample or syringe inlet but an additional connection between positions 4-5 or 5-6.

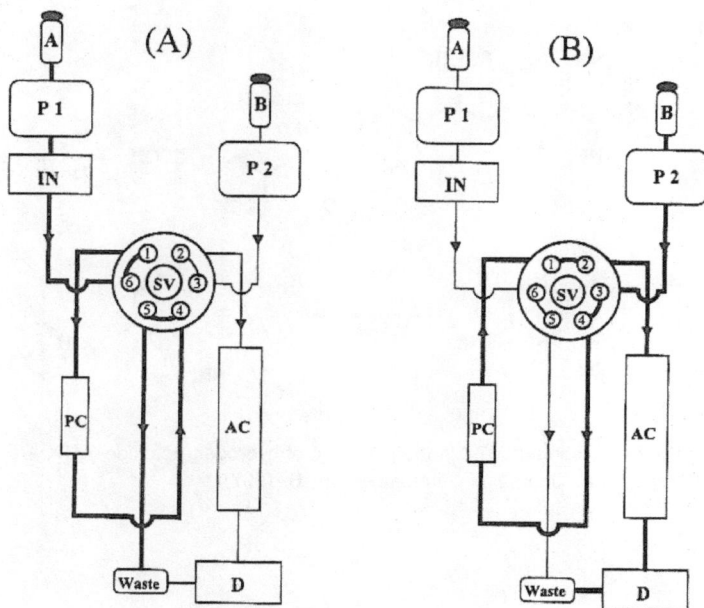

Figure 11: Schematic diagram of a column-switching system (AC=analytical column, P=pump, D=detector, SV=switching valve, A, B=mobile phases, IN=injector) (Manual LiChrospher® ADS, Merck)

For determination of *erythrocyte polyglutamates*, a HPLC method with post-column photo-oxidation was used [39].

By lowering the quantification and detection limit, post-column photo-oxidation followed by fluorimetric detection allows the measurement of nanomolar concentrations of MTX polyglutamates in erythrocytes.

Conversion of non-fluorescent MTX and its metabolites into fluorescent products was achieved by photo-oxidizing the analytes at 254 nm in the presence of hydrogen peroxide. The addition of hydrogen peroxide induces a chemical ring closure resulting in fluorescence (figure 12). In this process, the amount of oxidizer, irradiation time and the quality of reactor are determinants for the efficacy of the photoreaction [77].

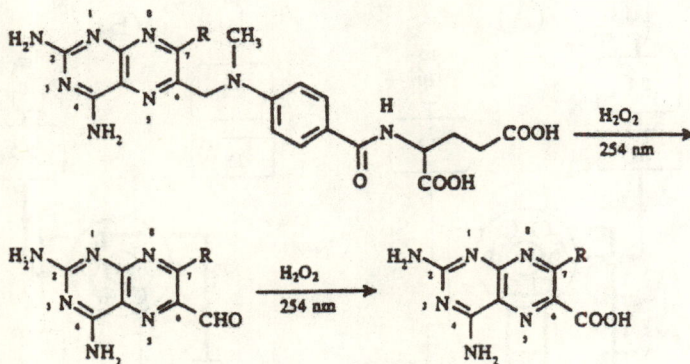

Figure 12: Photo-oxidation of MTX in the presence of hydrogen peroxide (MTX: R=H, 7-OH-MTX: R=OH) (Yu et al., Journal of Chromatography B, 1997)

3.2 MATERIALS AND METHODS

3.2.1 DETERMINATION OF PLASMA MTX AND 7-OH-MTX

3.2.1.1 Reagents and materials

Methotrexate (4-Amino-10-methylpteroylglutamic acid) was purchased from Schircks Laboratories (Jona, Switzerland). Acetonitrile (ACN) of gradient grade for Liquid Chromatography (LiChrosolv®) and ortho-phosphoric acid (85% p.a.) were obtained from Merck (Darmstadt, Germany). Sodium phosphate dibasic anhydrous, tetrabutylammonium hydroxide solution (TBAH, purissimum p.a. for ion chromatography) and hydrogen peroxide (H_2O_2, 30%, purum p.a.) were purchased from Fluka (Sigma Aldrich, Vienna, Austria). Biocoll® solution was purchased from Biochrom AG (Berlin, Germany). Millipore® water was used for making mobile phases.

Because 7-OH-MTX was not commercially available, its amount was calculated as an aliquot of MTX.

3.2.1.2 Preparation of standards and plasma samples

To avoid absorption of MTX to glassware, all solutions were kept in micro test-tubes (Eppendorf®, Hamburg, Germany). For protection of light, tubes were covered with aluminum foil.

Blank human plasma was obtained from the Department of Internal Medicine 1 at the Medical University of Vienna.

For measurement of intra-assay variability, different *standard solutions* in the range of 0 nM to 10000 nM were made. To prepare a 10000 nM solution, 10 µl of MTX stock solution (1 mg/ml) were diluted with plasma to the end volume of 2000 µl.

The standard curve contained the following concentrations:

- 10000 nM

- 5000 nM

- 2000 nM

- 1000 nM

- 500 nM

- 200 nM

- 150 nM

- 100 nM

- 50 nM

- 0 nM

Standard samples were prepared daily. Prior to injection, probes were centrifuged for 5 min at 6000 RPM to remove proteins and other particles. The injection volume was 100 µl.

Using the following formula, the relative centrifugal force (RCF) can be calculated:

$$RCF= \left(\frac{RPM}{1000}\right)^2 x\ r\ x\ 1.118$$

For preparation of rheumatoid arthritis *patient´s samples*, EDTA-whole blood (6 ml) was drawn and stored up to four hours at 4°C until further processing.

To process samples, 6 ml of Biocoll® solution were laid in a 15 ml conical tube before carefully adding 6 ml of EDTA-blood.

After a 20-min centrifugation step (1600 RPM, 4°C) to separate plasma from buffy coat (leukocytes and platelets) and RBCs (figure 13), plasma was stored at -80°C until HPLC analysis. Corresponding to standard samples, patient samples were centrifuged for 5 min at 6000 RPM prior to injection. The injection volume was 100 µl.

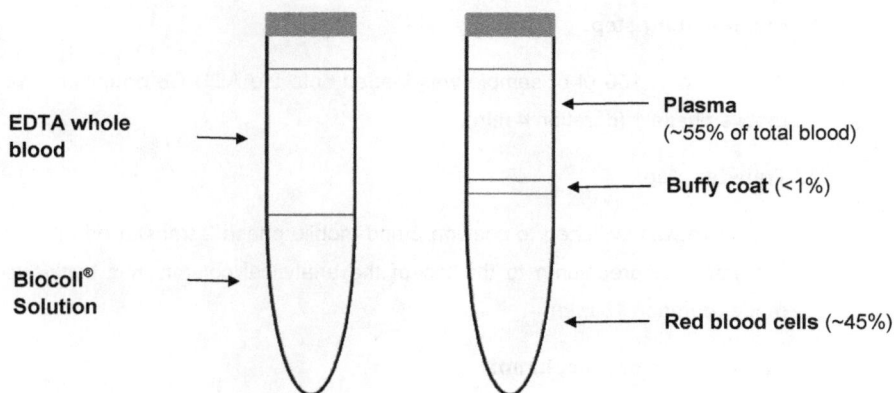

Figure 13: Ficoll Hyperpaque technique to separate plasma from buffy coat and RBCs

3.2.1.3   Chromatographic instrumentation and conditions

Studies were performed on an Agilent 1100 HPLC Chemstation system consisting of a binary pump, an autoinjector, a fluorimetric detector and a system controller. An external pump (Gilson®) was used to transport mobile phase 1 for loading plasma samples onto the precolumn. For post-column photo-oxidation, a photochemical reactor unit, equipped with a 254 nm low-pressure mercury UV-lamp and a 1/16-inch (o.d.) teflon tubing (0.25 mm i.d.) (Aura Industries, New York, USA), was implemented between the analytical column and the fluorimetric detector.

Chromatographic separation was performed on a LiChroCART® 250-4 LiChrospher® 100 RP-18 endcapped column (5 μm particle size, Merck), protected by a guard column (LiChroCART® 4-4 LiChrospher® 100 RP-18 endcapped (5 μm, Merck)). Additionally, a C8-alkyl-diol-silica (ADS) precolumn (LiChroCART® 25-4 LiChrospher® RP-8, Merck) was used for the column-switching system.

Using a column-switching system, the switching times had to be defined.

1. **Fractionating step:**

   At position 1, 100 µl of sample was loaded onto the ADS C8 precolumn with mobile phase 1 (duration 4 min).

2. **Transfer step:**

   The valve was switched to position 2 and mobile phase 2 transferred the analyte from the precolumn to the top of the analytical column in a back-flush mode (duration 18 min).

3. **Equilibration of precolumn:**

   The valve switched back to position 1 to equilibrate the precolumn with mobile phase 1. A new analysis cycle was started after 26 min.

Mobile phase 1, used for loading of the plasma sample onto the precolumn, consisted of 2 mM TBAH in phosphate buffer pH 7.4 with 2% ACN (50 mM).

1 L of mobile phase 1 was produced in the following way:

- 7.1 g Sodium phosphate dibasic anhydrous

- 1.3 ml TBAH

- 20 ml ACN

- pH adjustment with ortho-phosphoric acid (85% p.a.)

- Millipore® water ad 1000 ml

Mobile phase 2, used for the transfer and separation procedure, consisted of 5 mM TBAH and 0.2% H_2O_2 in 50 mM phosphate buffer pH 7.4.

1 L of mobile phase 2 was produced in the following way:

- 7.1 g Sodium phosphate dibasic anhydrous

- 3.3 ml TBAH

- 2 ml H_2O_2 (30% in water)

- pH adjustment with ortho-phosphoric acid (85% p.a.)

- Millipore® water ad 1000 ml

Mobile phase 3, the organic amount, consisted of 100% ACN.

After sterile filtration and degasing in an ultrasonic bath for 10 min, mobile phases were used at a flow rate of 1.0 ml/min. For optimization of separation, the ratio of mobile phase 2 and ACN (mobile phase 3) was 84:16.

Using fluorimetric detection, MTX and 7-OH-MTX were measured at an excitation wavelength set at 370 nm and an emission wavelength set at 417 nm. The fluorimetric signal of MTX was recorded at 13.8 min. The signal of 7-hydroxymethotrexate was measured at 15.3 min.

The chromatography was performed at ambient temperature.

A new analysis cycle was started after 26 min.

3.2.2 DETERMINATION OF ERYTHROCYTE MTX POLYGLUTA-MATES

3.2.2.1 Reagents and materials

Methotrexate (4-Amino-10-methylpteroylglutamic acid, MTXPG1), MTXPG2 (4-Amino-10-methylpteroyldiglutamic acid), MTXPG3 (4-Amino-10-methylpteroyltri-glutamic acid), MTXPG4 (4-Amino-10-methylpteroyltetraglutamic acid), MTXPG5 (4-Amino-10-methylpteroylpentaglutamic acid), MTXPG6 (4-Amino-10-methylpteroyl-hexaglutamic acid) and MTXPG7 (4-Amino-10-methylpteroylheptaglutamic acid) were purchased from Schircks Laboratories (Jona, Switzerland) as ammonium salts.

Acetonitrile (ACN) of gradient grade for Liquid Chromatography (LiChrosolv®), ammonium acetate (p.a.) and acetic acid (glacial) were obtained from Merck (Darmstadt, Germany). Hydrogen peroxide (H_2O_2 30%, purum p.a.) was purchased from Fluka (Sigma Aldrich, Vienna, Austria). Biocoll® solution and HBSS-solution were purchased from Biochrom AG (Berlin, Germany). Millipore® water was used for making mobile phases.

3.2.2.2 Preparation of standards and patient´s samples

To avoid absorption of MTX and MTXPGs to glassware, all solutions were kept in micro test-tubes (Eppendorf®, Hamburg, Germany). For protection of light, tubes were covered with aluminum foil.

For preparation of standard solutions in water, Millipore® water was used.

To measure intra-assay variability in water, different *standard solutions* in the range of 0 nM to 200 nM were made. For preparation of a 200 nM solution of MTXPG1-7, stock solutions of 10 µg/ml in H_2O were used.

Because of differences in molecular weight, the production of a 200 nM equimolar solution of MTXPG1-7 (total volume 10 ml) needed:

- 100.0 µl MTXPG1 stock solution (MW: 454.5)

- 125.0 µl MTXPG2 stock solution (MW: 634.7)

- 153.8 µl MTXPG3 stock solution (MW: 780.8)

- 181.8 µl MTXPG4 stock solution (MW: 926.9)

- 222.2 µl MTXPG5 stock solution (MW: 1073.1)

- 250.0 µl MTXPG6 stock solution (MW: 1219.2)

- 285.8 µl MTXPG7 stock solution (MW: 1365.4)

- 8681.4 µl of water

The standard curve contained the following concentrations:

- 200 nM

- 150 nM

- 100 nM

- 50 nM

- 20 nM

- 10 nM

- 0 nM

Standard samples were stored at -80°C and were stable for at least 12 months at these conditions. The injection volume was 80 µl.

For preparation of rheumatoid arthritis *patient's samples*, EDTA-whole blood (6 ml) was drawn and stored up to four hours at 4°C until further processing.

As previously described for preparation of plasma samples, 6 ml of Biocoll® solution were laid in a 15 ml conical tube before carefully adding 6 ml of EDTA-blood, using a pipette.

To separate plasma from buffy coat and RBCs (figure 13), samples were centrifuged for 20 min at 1600 RPM, 4°C. RBCs were washed twice in 3 volumes of HBSS-solution. After vortexing for 15 seconds, RBCs were centrifuged for 10 min at 1000 RPM each time. The supernatant was discarded.

In the next step, packed RBCs were hemolyzed with 3 volumes of water (12 ml) and vortexed for 15 seconds.

Probes were aliquoted in 1 ml tubes and boiled for 10 min at 100°C, using a dry block.

After boiling to denature proteins, cells were immediately put on ice for 15 min and finally centrifuged for 15 min at 3000 RPM (4°C).

The precipitate was discarded. The supernatant was aliquoted in 1 ml tubes and stored at -80°C until analysis.

After thawing and prior to injection, patient samples were centrifuged for 5 min at 15000 RPM. The injection volume was 80 µl.

3.2.2.3   Chromatographic instrumentation and conditions

Studies were performed on an Agilent 1100 HPLC Chemstation system consisting of a binary pump, an autoinjector, a fluorimetric detector and a system controller. For post-column photo-oxidation, a photochemical reactor unit equipped with a 254 nm low-pressure mercury UV-lamp and a 1/16-inch (o.d.) teflon tubing (0.25 mm i.d.)

(Aura Industries, New York, USA) was implemented between the analytical column and the fluorimetric detector.

For chromatographic separation, a LiChroCART® 250-4 LiChrospher® 100 RP-18 endcapped column (5 µm particle size, Merck), protected by a LiChroCART® 4-4 LiChrospher® 100 RP-18 endcapped guard column (5 µm, Merck) was used.

Mobile phase 1 consisted of 10 mM ammonium acetate (pH 6.50), containing 2% of hydrogen peroxide (30% in water).

1 L of mobile phase 1 was produced in the following way:

- 0.77 g Ammonium acetate

- 2 ml H_2O_2 (30% in water)

- pH adjustment with acetic acid (glacial)

- Millipore® water ad 1000 ml

Mobile phase 2 consisted of 100% ACN.

After sterile filtration, mobile phases were used at a flow rate of 1.0 ml per min.

For optimization of separation, a 17-min linear gradient from 0% to 17% ACN (mobile phase 2) was used. After 17 min, the mobile phase was returned to 100% mobile phase 1 until the stop time of 22 min. Before starting the next analysis cycle, the system was re-equilibrated for 15 min (post-time).

Using fluorimetric detection, MTXPGs were measured at an excitation wavelength set at 274 nm and an emission wavelength set at 470 nm. The fluorimetric signals of MTXPGs were recorded between 7.00 and 14.10 min.

The chromatography was performed at ambient temperature.

3.3 RESULTS

3.3.1 CALIBRATION CURVES AND INTRA-ASSAY VARIABILITY

3.3.1.1 Intra-assay variability of MTX and 7-OH-MTX in plasma

Because an already published HPLC method was used, inter-assay variability of MTX and 7-OH-MTX in plasma was not performed.

Intra-day precision was determined by analyzing 10 different concentrations of MTX in plasma (0, 50, 100, 150, 200, 500, 1000, 2000, 5000 and 10000 nM) using replications on 5 subsequent days. Imprecision was defined by estimating the coefficient of variation (CV) in %. Results are shown in table 7.

Concentration	Mean Area (LU*s)	SD	CV (%)	Injection #
0 nM	-	-	-	5
50 nM	3.64	0.21	5.70	5
100 nM	6.10	0.19	3.16	5
150 nM	8.79	0.14	1.60	5
200 nM	11.49	0.58	5.07	5
500 nM	27.54	0.16	0.59	5
1000 nM	60.17	2.96	4.93	5
2000 nM	112.05	3.53	3.15	5
5000 nM	252.80	4.92	1.94	5
10000 nM	478.19	28.31	5.92	5

Table 7: Intra-assay variability of MTX in plasma (CV= coefficient of variation in %, SD=standard deviation)

The calibration curve of MTX in plasma demonstrated a linear relationship between peak area and concentration with a correlation coefficient of 0.999 (figure 14).

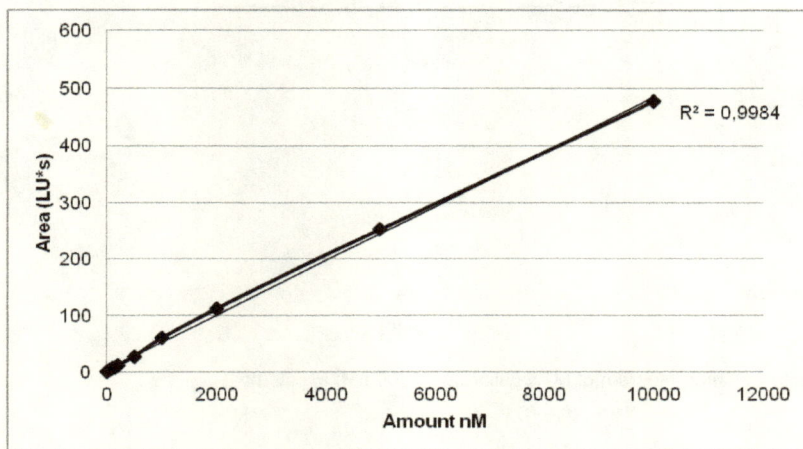

Figure 14: Calibration curve of MTX in plasma

7-OH-MTX was not commercially available and therefore not included in calibration curves. As a consequence, 7-OH-MTX was calculated as an aliquot of MTX for analyzing patient's samples.

The limit of detection, defined as the concentration yielding a signal-to-noise-ratio of 2:1, was 53.87 nM for MTX.

Figure 15 shows a typical chromatogram of MTX calibrator in plasma (1000 nM).

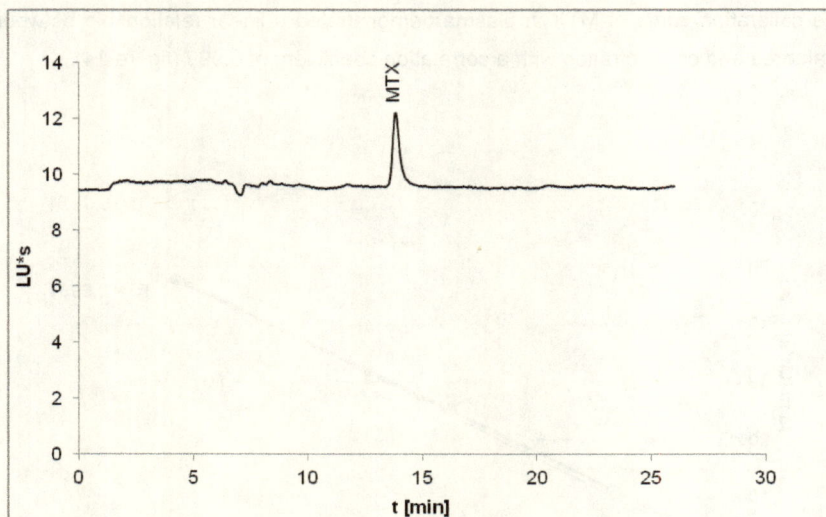

Figure 15: Chromatogram of MTX calibrator (1000 nM) in plasma

3.3.1.2 Intra-assay variability of MTX polyglutamates in water

Because a previously published HPLC method was used, inter-assay variability of MTX polyglutamates in water was not performed.

Intra-day precision was determined by analyzing 7 different concentrations of MTXPG1-7 in water (0, 10, 20, 50, 100, 150 and 200 nM), using replications on 5 subsequent days.

Imprecision was defined by estimating the coefficient of variation (CV) in %. Results are shown in table 8.

Calibrator	Concentration	Mean Area (LU*s)	SD	CV (%)	Injection #
MTXPG1	0 nM	-	-	-	5
	10 nM	37.56	0.04	0.10	5
	20 nM	71.64	0.20	0.28	5
	50 nM	174.51	0.58	0.33	5
	100 nM	359.21	0.18	0.05	5
	150 nM	489.30	0.90	0.18	5
	200 nM	736.43	0.89	0.12	5
MTXPG2	0 nM	-	-	-	5
	10 nM	31.59	0.20	0.62	5
	20 nM	59.42	0.15	0.26	5
	50 nM	149.19	1.02	0.68	5
	100 nM	308.49	1.97	0.64	5
	150 nM	424.91	5.57	1.31	5
	200 nM	631.85	0.91	0.14	5
MTXPG3	0 nM	-	-	-	5
	10 nM	21.47	0.10	0.44	5
	20 nM	40.00	0.20	0.49	5
	50 nM	106.35	0.29	0.27	5
	100 nM	217.45	0.18	0.08	5
	150 nM	310.13	1.36	0.44	5
	200 nM	445.38	0.94	0.21	5
MTXPG4	0 nM	-	-	-	5
	10 nM	22.62	0.21	0.93	5
	20 nM	40.08	0.18	0.45	5
	50 nM	114.35	0.33	0.29	5
	100 nM	232.49	0.79	0.34	5

Table 8a: Intra-assay variability of MTXPG1-7 in water (CV= coefficient of variation in %, SD=standard deviation)

Calibrator	Concentration	Mean Area (LU*s)	SD	CV (%)	Injection #
MTXPG4	150 nM	345.93	2.22	0.64	5
	200 nM	489.16	0.96	0.20	5
MTXPG5	0 nM	-	-	-	5
	10 nM	15.12	0.21	1.38	5
	20 nM	26.84	0.49	1.83	5
	50 nM	76.60	0.08	0.10	5
	100 nM	158.42	1.17	0.74	5
	150 nM	249.02	1.90	0.76	5
	200 nM	350.31	1.24	0.35	5
MTXPG6	0 nM	-	-	-	5
	10 nM	11.35	0.15	1.31	5
	20 nM	23.27	0.44	1.89	5
	50 nM	70.35	0.19	0.26	5
	100 nM	153.58	1.27	0.83	5
	150 nM	252.58	1.71	0.68	5
	200 nM	338.82	2.08	0.61	5
MTXPG7	0 nM	-	-	-	5
	10 nM	3.84	0.14	3.58	5
	20 nM	10.49	0.23	2.17	5
	50 nM	35.29	0.27	0.75	5
	100 nM	88.36	1.14	1.29	5
	150 nM	155.36	1.38	0.89	5
	200 nM	204.62	2.03	0.99	5

Table 8b: Intra-assay variability of MTXPG1-7 in water (CV= coefficient of variation in %, SD=standard deviation)

The calibration curves for MTXPG1-7 in water demonstrated a linear relationship between peak area and concentration with the following correlation coefficients (figures 16-22).

- MTXPG1: 0.997
- MTXPG2: 0.997
- MTXPG3: 0.999
- MTXPG4: 0.999
- MTXPG5: 0.999
- MTXPG6: 0.999
- MTXPG7: 0.996

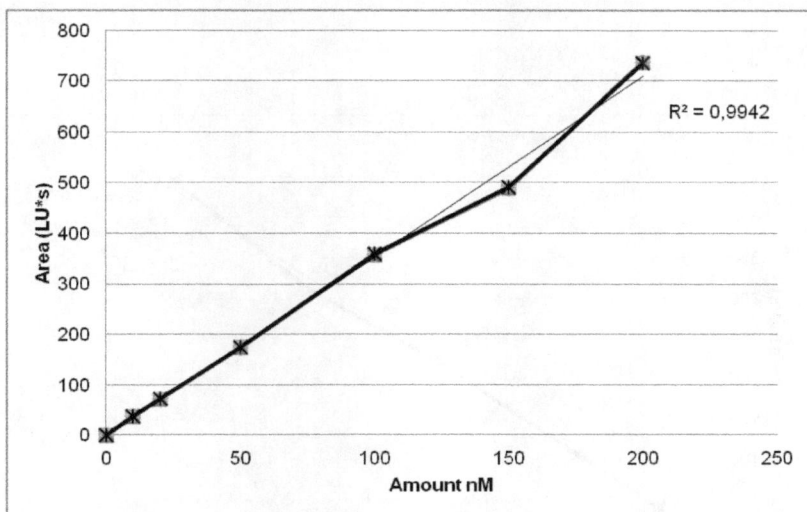

Figure 16: Calibration curve of MTPG1 in water

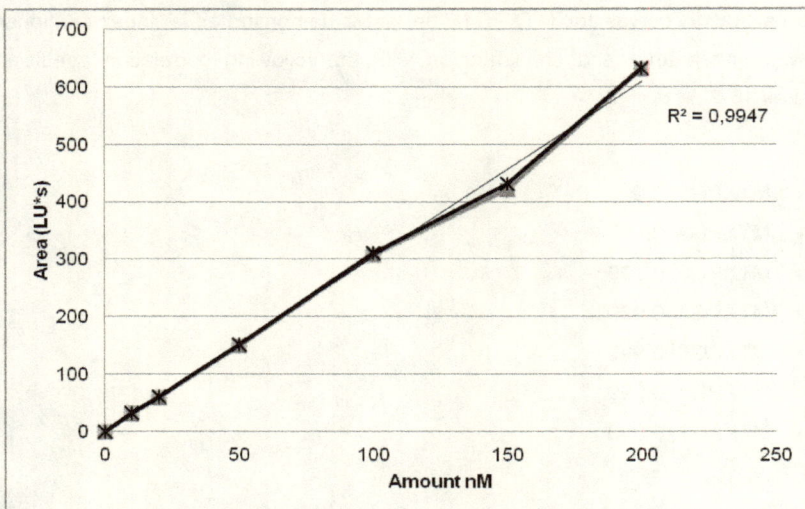

Figure 17: Calibration curve of MTPG2 in water

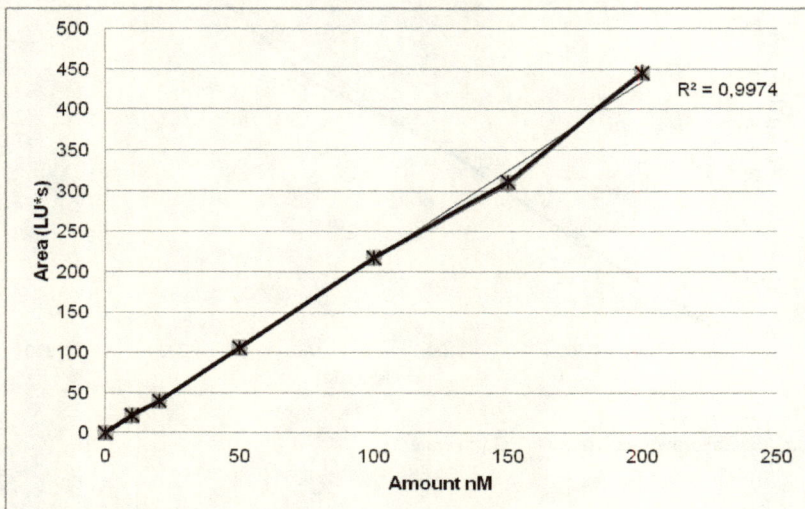

Figure 18: Calibration curve of MTPG3 in water

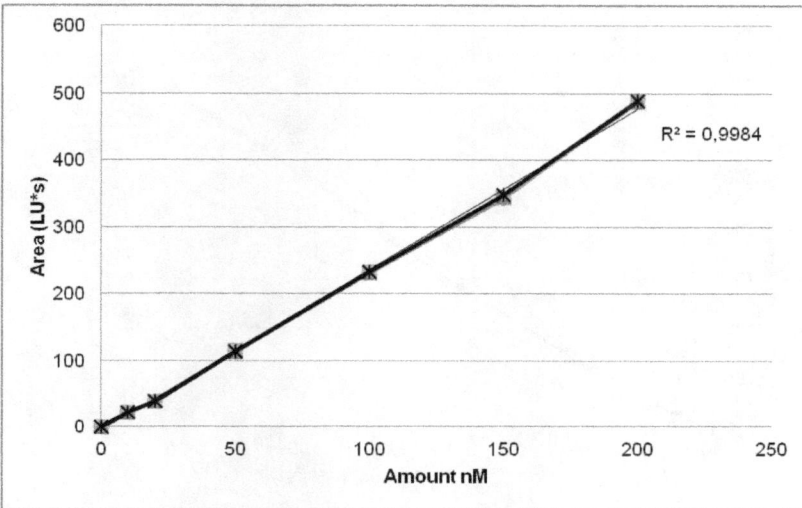

Figure 19: Calibration curve of MTPG4 in water

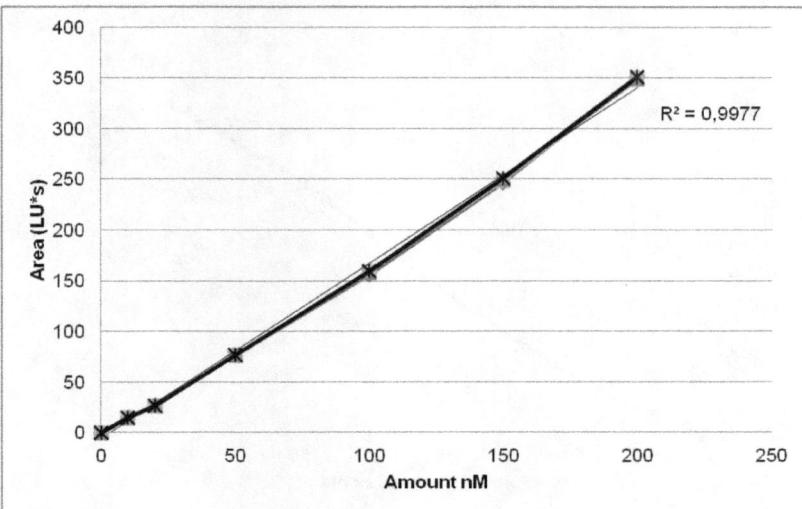

Figure 20: Calibration curve of MTPG5 in water

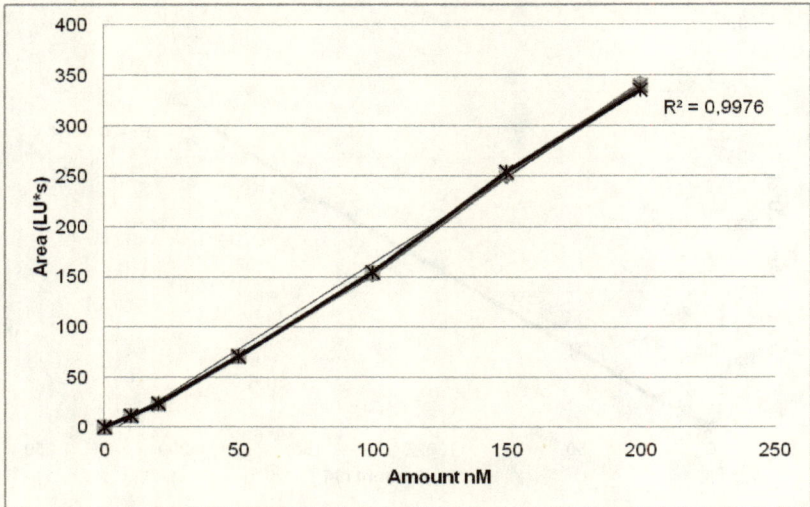

Figure 21: Calibration curve of MTPG6 in water

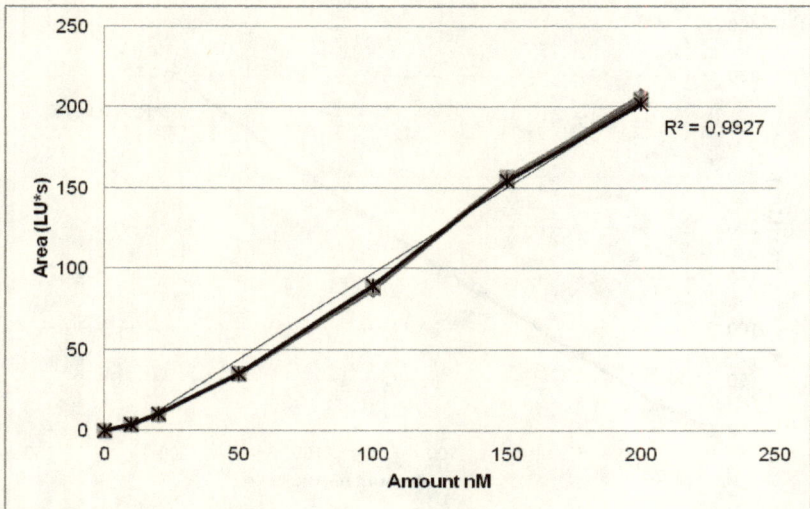

Figure 22: Calibration curve of MTPG7 in water

A typical chromatogram of MTXPG1-7 calibrators in water (20 nM) is shown in figure 23.

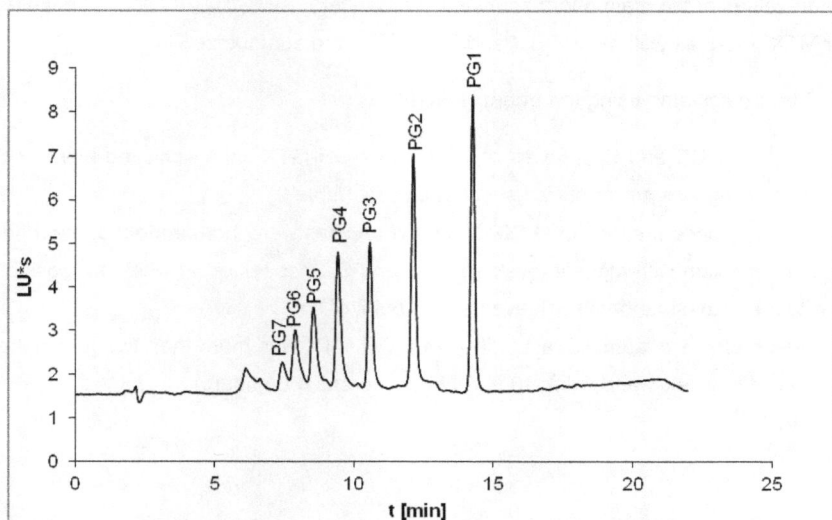

Figure 23: Chromatogram of MTXPG1-7 calibrators (20 nM) in water

Because of differences in ring closure and consequently in the intensity of fluorescence, the limit of detection was 0.37 nM for MTXPG1, 0.52 nM for MTXPG2, 2 nM for MTXPG3, 5 nM for MTXPG4, 13 nM for MTXPG5, 28 nM for MTXPG6 and 48 nM for MTXPG7.

3.3.2 PHARMACOKINETIC ANALYSIS OF MTX, 7-OH-MTX AND MTXPGS IN PATIENTS

Mean values of the main pharmacokinetic parameters (AUC, T_{max}, C_{max}, and half-life) for MTXPG1-3 as well as for MTX and 7-OH-MTX are summarized in table 9.

AUC was calculated using the trapezoidal rule.

The highest AUC and C_{max} levels of MTX and 7-OH-MTX were achieved at week 5, when the drug was administered subcutaneously (table 9).

In contrast, concentrations of MTXPGs in erythrocytes were independent of the mode of administration with highest levels of AUC and C_{max} observed at week 10, possibly due to a steady-state being achieved at this point of time.

At week 5 after s.c. administration, T_{max} of 7-OH-MTX was more than two-fold higher compared to week 1 and week 10 (8.63 hours versus 4.00 hours).

	AUC (nM*h)	T_{max} (h)	C_{max} (nM)	Half-life (h)
MTXPG1				
Week 1	2964 (± 5578)	12.11 (± 37.77)	17.42 (± 8.37)	346.72 (± 609.02)
Week 5	12734 (± 11683)	3.61 (± 0.94)	40.92 (± 12.21)	649.45 (± 611.06)
Week 10	53001 (± 1.21E5)	3.74 (± 0.79)	41.87 (± 10.57)	1883.75 (± 3406.73)
MTXPG2				
Week 1	474 (± 457)	132.50 (± 66.85)	11.06 (± 12.51)	-
Week 5	49145 (± 1.40E5)	111.61 (± 78.62)	15.92 (± 3.99)	7705.19 (± 10373.71)
Week 10	8260 (± 14340)	75.47 (± 78.22)	22.06 (± 5.61)	1452.18 (± 855.82)
MTXPG3				
Week 1	9925 (± 12607)	84.58 (± 87.13)	45.43 (± 37.69)	324.13 (± 234.00)
Week 5	15655 (± 23258)	105.21 (± 78.77)	48.36 (± 34.76)	487.29 (± 94.65)
Week 10	90655 (± 1.88E5)	55.89 (± 65.23)	68.67 (± 36.45)	1801.88 (± 1727.01)
MTX				
Week 1	9756 (± 5665)	2.03 (± 1.05)	620.22 (± 397.79)	5.44 (± 7.34)
Week 5	24132 (± 40982)	2.03 (± 1.05)	772.34 (± 301.64)	22.25 (± 55.08)
Week 10	11098 (± 5812)	1.63 (± 0.57)	721.14 (± 384.28)	8.63 (± 15.93)
7-OH-MTX				
Week 1	44727 (± 33716)	4.00 (± 0.00)	1043.78 (± 765.99)	63.61 (± 48.06)
Week 5	54153 (± 34893)	8.63 (± 13.87)	1129.06 (± 667.07)	39.30 (± 18.93)
Week 10	46930 (± 28363)	4.00 (± 0.00)	1125.90 (± 821.10)	41.81 (± 23.84)

Table 9: Pharmacokinetics of MTX, 7-OH-MTX and MTXPG1-3: results are expressed as the mean (SD)

Unfortunately, interferences occurred at the chromatographic positions of MTXPG4 and MTXPG5, so that these polyglutamates could not be interpreted.

First, this phenomenon may be explained by the fact that long-chained MTX-polyglutamates are structural analogs of folic acid and therefore the system possibly was not selective enough to differentiate between natural occurring folates and MTX-polyglutamates.

A second explanation could be that PG4 and PG5 may occur naturally in humans, even though this is highly improbable.

For clarification, some additional studies e.g. co-chromatography of MTXPG4 and MTXPG5 were performed, which are described at the end of chapter 3.

Nevertheless, this problem could not be solved satisfactorily during the thesis project.

MTXPG6 and MTXPG7 were below the limit of detection in the presented population of rheumatoid arthritis patients, which is in accordance to other clinical trials [39].

Figure 24 illustrates a blank RBC sample. In figure 25, a typical patient's chroma-togram of erythrocyte MTX polyglutamates is shown, representing a sample taken 1.5 hours after MTX intake.

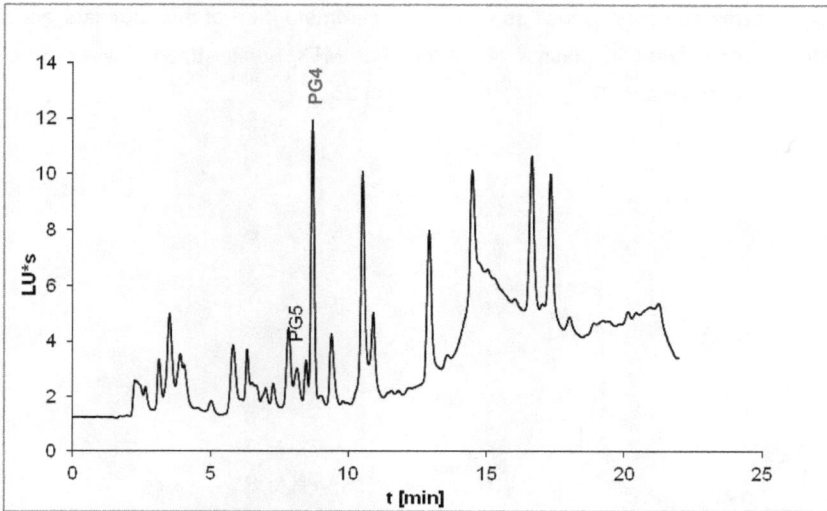

Figure 24: Chromatogram of a blank RBC sample

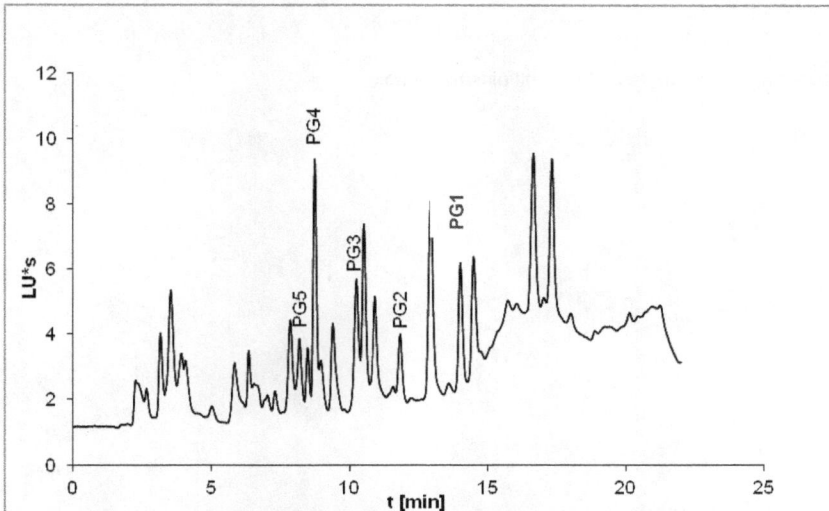

Figure 25: Patient's chromatogram of a RBC sample (Week 10, 1.5 h after MTX intake)

Blank plasma samples as well as a patient's chromatogram of methotrexate and 7-hydroxymethotrexate in plasma (4 hours after MTX administration, week 5) are shown in figure 26 and 27.

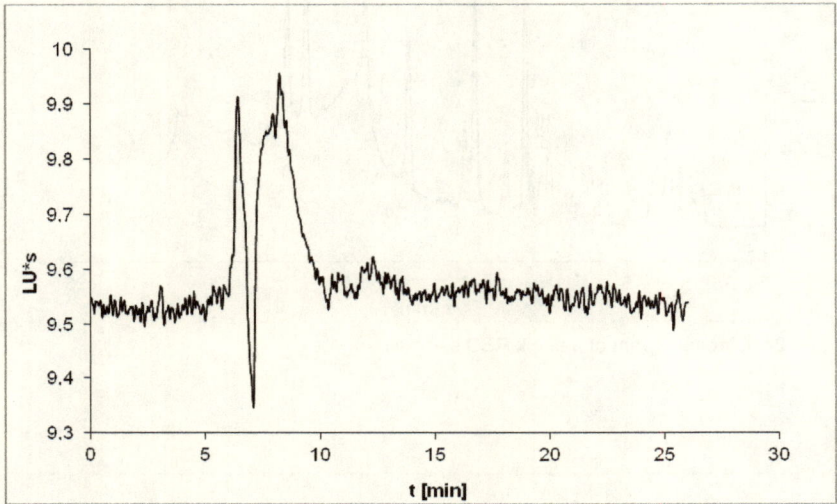

Figure 26: Chromatogram of a blank plasma sample

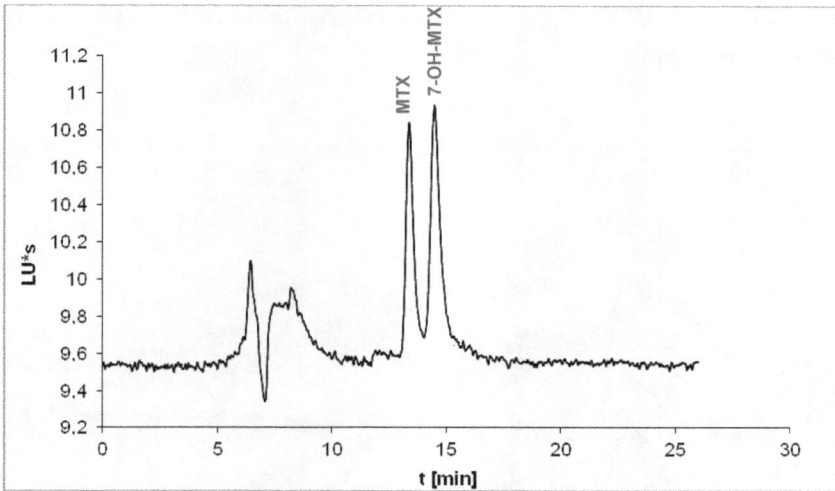

Figure 27: Chromatogram of a patient´s plasma sample (Week 5, 4 h after MTX intake)

The complete pharmacokinetic profile of methotrexate and its metabolites for 16 weeks is presented in figure 28.

The illustration points up, that plasma MTX is completely eliminated within 48 hours after drug administration. 7-OH-MTX, the main metabolite formed in the liver and associated with side effects, is detectable over a period of one week after taking MTX with T_{max} levels of 4 hours.

Formation of erythrocyte polyglutamates MTXPG2 and MTXPG3 starts simultaneously within one week after beginning methotrexate therapy. This may indicate the distribution of methotrexate from plasma to intracellular storage sites, for example to erythrocytes.

Interestingly, before the second administration a redistribution of MTXPG1 to plasma was observed 168 hours after MTX intake, even though serum MTX was totally excreted by the kidneys within 48 hours. This phenomenon may be explained by a saturation mechanism of erythrocytes.

73

For MTXPG4 and MTXPG5, no relevant changes in concentration were observed after drug administration.

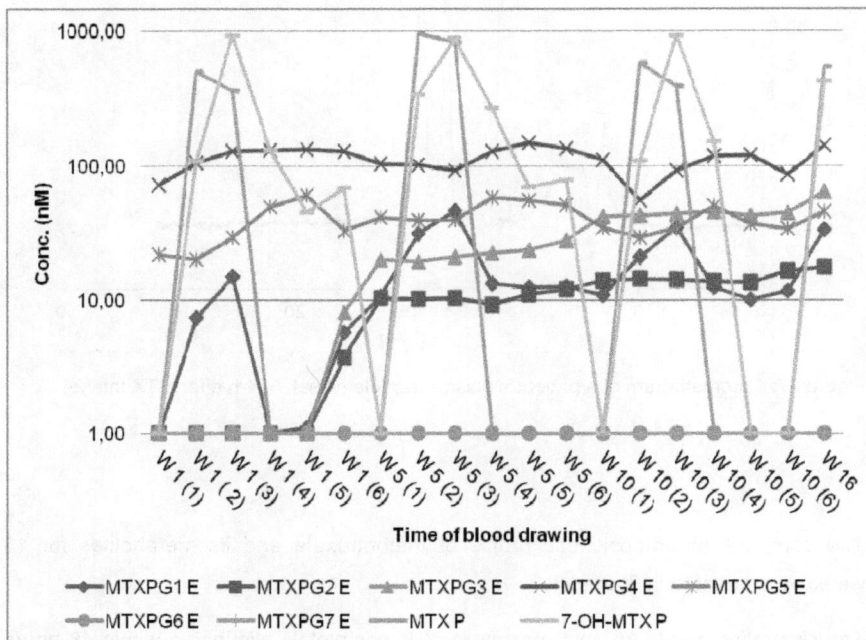

Figure 28: Pharmacokinetic profile of MTX administered for 16 weeks (W=week, E=erythrocyte, P=plasma, 1=blank sample, 2=1.5 h after MTX, 3=4 h after MTX, 4=48 h after MTX, 5=96 h after MTX, 6=168 h after MTX) (logarithmic scale)

3.3.2.1   Correlation of pharmacokinetic and clinical parameters

a) Comparison of a standard and a higher starting dose

Considering clinical parameters, the original thought that a higher starting dose of MTX possibly has a faster onset of action than a standard dose did not prove true.

However, at week 1 pharmacokinetic analysis of MTX, 7-OH-MTX and erythrocyte polyglutamates showed statistically significant differences between the two different dosing schemata (Mann-Whitney-U-test for independent samples, significance level 0.05). C_{max} (nM) levels of erythrocyte MTXPG1 and of serum MTX were statistically significant higher when starting with 25 mg MTX (figure 29 and 30).

At week 5, the use of the Mann-Whitney-U-test for independent samples showed no significant differences in the pharmacokinetic parameters (AUC, C_{max}, T_{max}) of MTXPG1-3, comparing the different dosing schemata.

Results of the Mann-Whitney-U-test for independent samples are presented in table 10.

Parameter	Standard dose	High dose	Significance
Week 1			
MTXPG1 AUC (nM*h)	4054 (± 7691)	1751 (± 552)	0.072
MTXPG1 T_{max} (h)	19.90 (± 52.05)	3.44 (± 1.10)	0.633
MTXPG1 C_{max} (nM)	12.81 (± 3.30)	22.54 (± 9.44)	**0.003***
MTXPG2 AUC (nM*h)	513 (± 402)	435 (± 532)	0.248
MTXPG2 T_{max} (h)	147.50 (± 57.98)	117.50 (± 75.50)	0.269
MTXPG2 C_{max} (nM)	7.01 (± 4.17)	15.11 (±16.76)	0.916
MTXPG3 AUC (nM*h)	11934 (± 11952)	8490 (± 13797)	0.465
MTXPG3 T_{max} (h)	101.10 (± 91.61)	72.79 (± 89.07)	0.662
MTXPG3 C_{max} (nM)	56.31 (± 47.11)	37.66 (± 30.91)	0.515
MTX AUC (nM*h)	7483 (± 4100)	12282 (± 6297)	**0.050***
MTX T_{max} (h)	2.25 (± 1.21)	1.78 (± 0.83)	0.326
MTX C_{max} (nM)	422.66 (± 181.57)	839.74 (± 464.69)	**0.022***
MTX half-life (h)	7.47 (± 10.37)	3.67 (± 2.81)	0.908
7-OH-MTX AUC (nM*h)	31818 (± 26608)	59071 (± 36351)	0.060
7-OH-MTX T_{max} (h)	4.00 (± 0.00)	4.00 (± 0.00)	1.000
7-OH-MTX C_{max} (nM)	858.68 (± 617.31)	1249.45 (± 895.01)	0.327
7-OH-MTX half-life (h)	70.52 (± 43.87)	59.01 (± 52.72)	0.724
Week 5			
MTXPG1 AUC (nM*h)	9567 (± 8544)	16253 (± 14090)	0.327
MTXPG1 T_{max} (h)	3.25 (± 1.05)	4.00 (± 0.00)	0.081
MTXPG1 C_{max} (nM)	38.56 (± 11.33)	43.55 (± 13.29)	0.327
MTXPG2 AUC (nM*h)	32325 (± 73452)	67835 (± 1.93E5)	0.414
MTXPG2 T_{max} (h)	101.25 (± 86.18)	123.11 (± 72.60)	0.603
MTXPG2 C_{max} (nM)	16.16 (± 3.22)	15.67 (± 4.90)	0.683
MTXPG3 AUC (nM*h)	18494 (± 26429)	12501 (± 20249)	0.935
MTXPG3 T_{max} (h)	94.30 (± 82.62)	117.33 (± 77.25)	0.649
MTXPG3 C_{max} (nM)	48.06 (± 39.94)	48.69 (± 30.39)	0.514

Table 10: Between-group-comparison of pharmacokinetic parameters of a standard and a higher starting dose at week 1 and week 5 (Mann-Whitney-U-test for independent samples, significance level 0.05): results are expressed as the mean (SD)

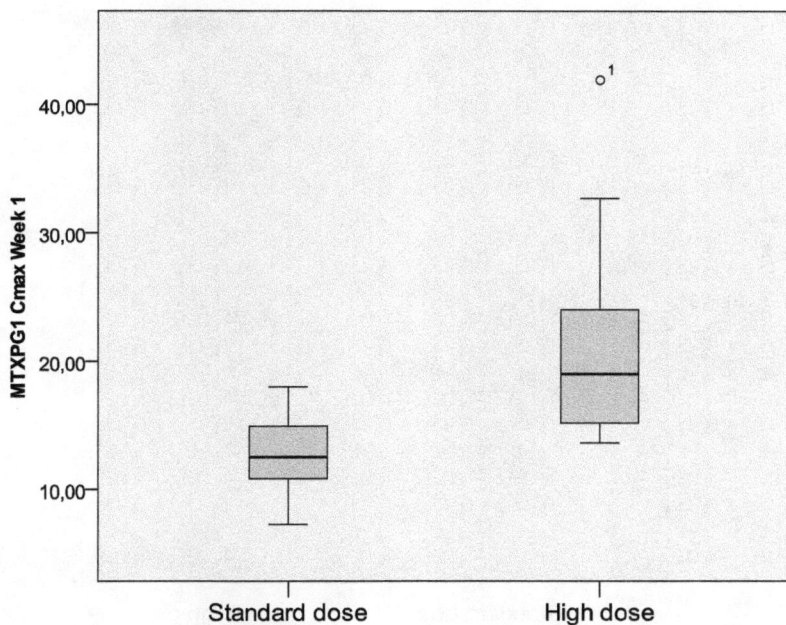

Figure 29: Box-and-Whisker plot MTXPG1 in erythrocytes: C_{max} (nM) at week 1 (Comparison Standard and High-dose), values given as the median with 25th and 75th percentiles; min, max

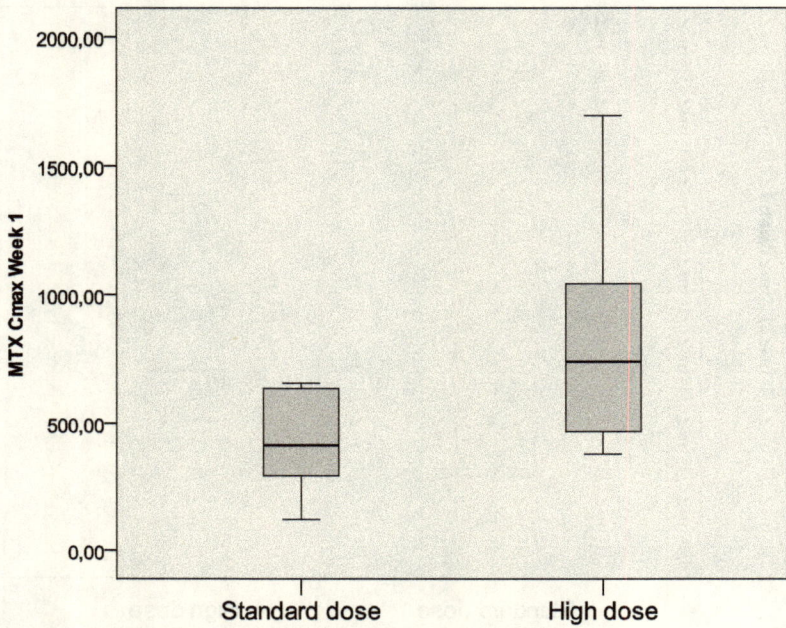

Figure 30: Box-and-Whisker plot serum MTX: C_{max} (nM) at week 1 (Comparison Standard and High-dose), values given as the median with 25th and 75th percentiles; min, max

b) Comparison of oral and subcutaneous administration

To compare the pharmacokinetics and efficacy of oral and subcutaneous methotrexate administration, each patient received a s.c. dose of 25 mg MTX at week 5. Therefore, a direct comparison with week 10, where 25 mg MTX were administered orally, was possible. Table 11 shows that C_{max} levels of MTXPG2 and MTXPG3 are significantly higher at week 10 compared to week 5, which is likely due to the fact that steady-state is not achieved before week 10 (Wilcoxon-test for paired samples, significance level 0.05). For plasma MTX, no significant differences were observed.

Parameter	Week 5 s.c.	Week 10 p.o.	Significance
MTX C_{max} (nM)	772.34 (± 301.64)	721.14 (± 384.28)	0.809
MTXPG2 C_{max} (nM)	15.92 (± 3.99)	22.06 (± 5.61)	< 0.001
MTXPG3 C_{max} (nM)	48.36 (± 34.76)	68.67 (± 36.45)	< 0.001

Table 11: Comparison of subcutaneous and oral MTX administration: Wilcoxon-test for paired samples, significance level 0.05; results are expressed as the mean (SD)

Further, this study confirms the inter-patient variability of clinical response in patients receiving methotrexate (see table 9, standard deviations). Pharmacokinetic results do not indicate a significant benefit of a subcutaneous MTX administration. No relevant differences in clinics as well as in MTX and 7-hydroxymethotrexate plasma levels were observed.

Nevertheless, in individual cases – for example in MTX non-responders after oral administration - the subcutaneous administration of methotrexate may be the last resort to reduce rheumatoid arthritis symptoms before switching to biologicals.

c) Correlation of pharmacokinetics and pharmacodynamics

To analyze the impact of serum MTX and MTXPGs erythrocyte levels on clinical parameters, correlation analysis calculating the Spearman´s as well as the Pearson´s coefficient was performed.

At week 5, C_{max} of MTXPG1 (nM) negatively correlated with monocytes (-0.507, p=0.027), which play an essential role as inflammatory parameters in rheumatoid arthritis.

It could be shown, that MTXPG2 is a potential marker for clinical outcome in rheumatoid arthritis. At week 5, a statistically significant positive correlation of MTXPG2 C_{max} levels and improvement in DAS-28 (+0.518, p=0.023) was noted. In addition, a negative correlation between C_{max} levels of MTXPG2 and eosinophils was observed (-0.559, p=0.013). Elevated levels of eosinophils are a typical characteristic for rheumatoid arthritis.

In contrast, high levels of MTXPG3 could have a negative impact on inflammatory markers. This is particularly evident because there was a statistically significant positive correlation between C_{max} levels of MTXPG3 and ESR (+0.505, p=0.027) as well as CRP (+0.627, p=0.004).

Reflecting the typical pharmacokinetics of methotrexate, the formation of polyglutamates in erythrocytes negatively correlated with C_{max} of MTX in plasma. Further, a positive correlation between C_{max} of MTX and 7-OH-MTX is evident (+0.580, p=0.009).

Additionally, at week 10 C_{max} levels of MTXPG2 negatively correlated with basophils (-0.478, p=0.038) and eosinophils (-0.531, p=0.019) – both potentially inflammatory parameters involved in the disease. This observation could indicate a potential use for MTXPG2 as a marker for response of methotrexate in rheumatoid arthritis.

Statistically significant correlations are presented in table 12.

Pharmacokinetic parameter	Correlation partner	Correlation	Significance (two-sided)
Week 5			
MTXPG1 C_{max} (nM)	Leukocytes (/nl)	+ 0.564	0.012
	ANC (/nl)	+ 0.548	0.015
	Monocytes (%)	- 0.507	0.027
	MTXPG2 C_{max} (nM)	+ 0.507	0.027
MTXPG2 C_{max} (nM)	Improvement in DAS-28	+ 0.518	0.023
	Leukocytes (/nl)	+ 0.721	0.000
	ANC (/nl)	+ 0.669	0.002
	Eosinophils (%)	- 0.559	0.013
	MTXPG1 C_{max} (nM)	+ 0.507	0.027
	MTXPG2 AUC (nM*h)	+ 0.564	0.012
MTXPG3 C_{max} (nM)	ESR (mm/h)	+ 0.505	0.027
	CRP (mg/dl)	+ 0.627	0.004
	MTX C_{max} (nM)	- 0.483	0.036
	MTXPG3 AUC (nM*h)	+ 0.804	0.000
MTX C_{max} (nM)	MTXPG3 C_{max} (nM)	- 0.483	0.036
	7-OH-MTX C_{max} (nM)	+ 0.580	0.009
	MTXPG1 AUC (nM*h)	- 0.543	0.016
	MTXPG3 AUC (nM*h)	- 0.556	0.013
Week 10			
MTXPG1 C_{max} (nM)	MTXPG1 AUC (nM*h)	+ 0.488	0.034
	MTXPG2 C_{max} (nM)	+ 0.557	0.013
MTXPG2 C_{max} (nM)	Eosinophils (%)	- 0.531	0.019
	Basophils (%)	- 0.478	0.038
	MTXPG1 C_{max} (nM)	+ 0.557	0.013
	Improvement in DAS-28	+ 0.475	0.040*
MTX AUC (nM*h)	MTX C_{max} (nM)	+ 0.777	0.000
	7-OH-MTX AUC (nM*h)	+ 0.494	0.032
	7-OH-MTX C_{max} (nM)	+ 0.537	0.018

Table 12: Correlation analysis of pharmacokinetic and clinical parameters using Pearson's correlation coefficient (except *: Calculation using Spearman's correlation coefficient)

Figure 31 shows a scatter-plot of the positive correlation between C_{max} of MTXPG2 and improvement in DAS-28 at week 5. Figures 32 and 33 exemplify the negative correlations of C_{max} levels of MTXPG2 with basophils and eosinophils at week 10.

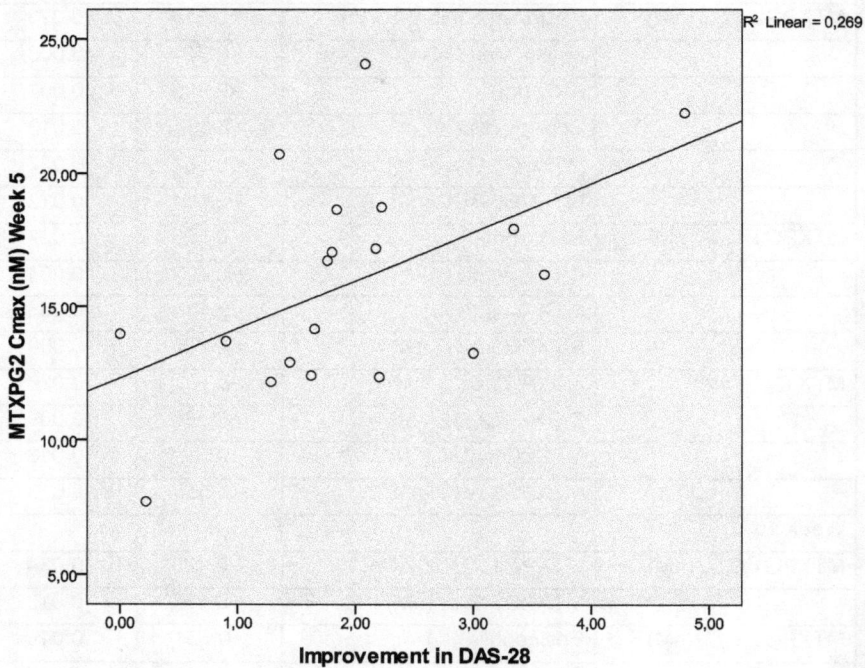

Figure 31: Scatter-plot: Correlation of MTXPG2 (C_{max}, nM) and improvement in DAS-28 at week 5

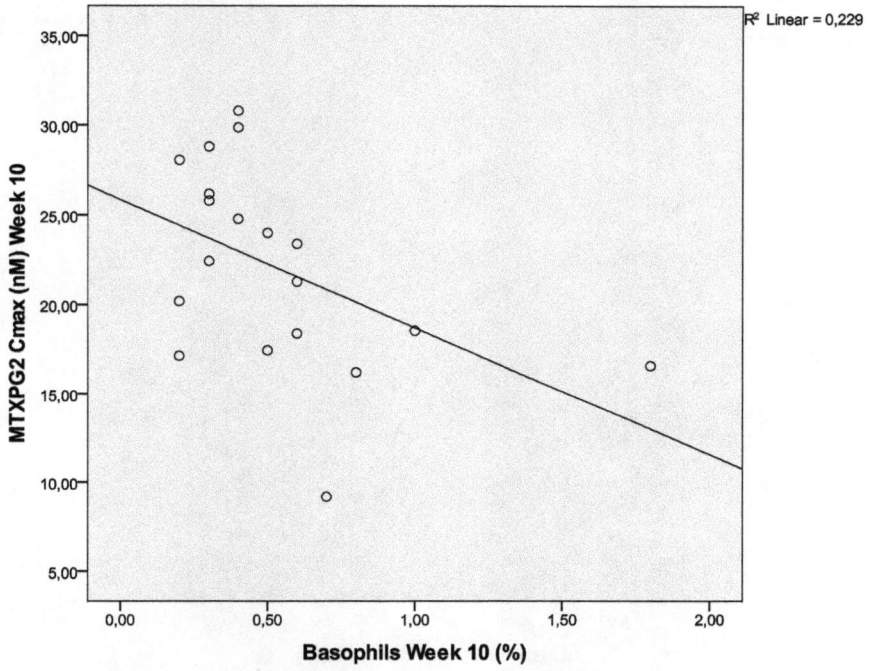

Figure 32: Scatter-plot: Correlation of MTXPG2 (C_{max}, nM) and basophils (%) at week 10

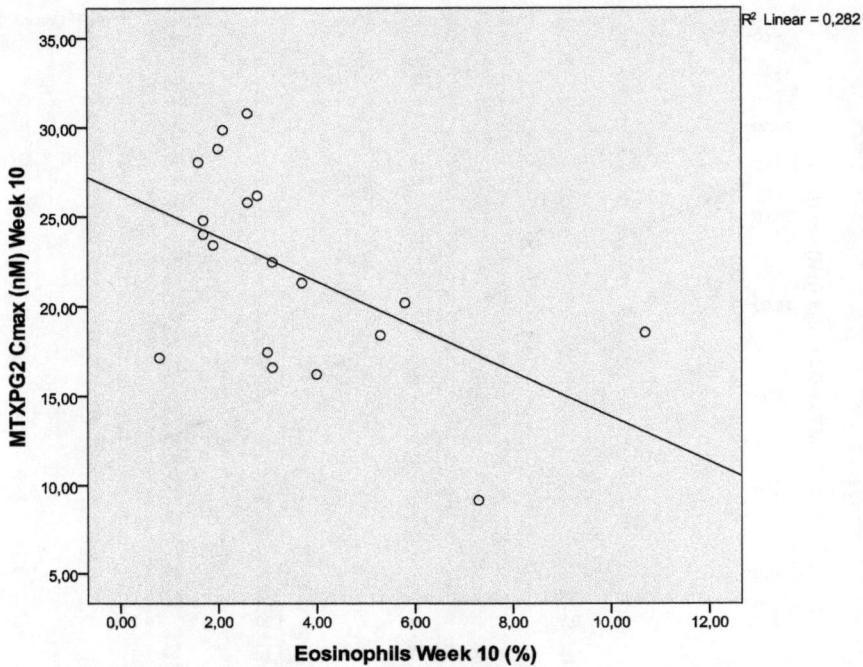

Figure 33: Scatter-plot: Correlation of MTXPG2 (C_{max}, nM) and eosinophils (%) at week 10

3.3.2.2   Additional studies

a) Optimization of the photochemical reaction

As previously described, photo-oxidation was required for conversion of non-fluorescent MTX and its metabolites into fluorescent products.

In addition to the amount of oxidizer (hydrogen peroxide), the irradiation time significantly contributes to the chemical reaction and determines the outcome of the oxidizing step. Irradiation time is influenced by the window size of the UV-lamp.

To find out the optimum conditions for the photochemical reaction, different window sizes were left open in the middle of the UV-lamp. The rest of the lamp was covered with aluminum foil on either side.

The following window sizes were tested by measuring peak areas of MTXPG1-7 (100 nM) with HPLC technique:

- Full length of the UV-lamp (without aluminum foil)

- 4 cm window

- 3 cm window

- 2 cm window

- 1 cm window

- 0.5 cm window

Interestingly, using 1- and 2-cm windows resulted in maximum peak areas of MTXPGs. Areas of MTXPG1-3 were highest using the 1-cm window, areas of all other polyglutamates (MTXPG4-7) achieved their maximum when operating with the 2-cm window (figure 34).

Because MTXPG6 and MTXPG7 have never been detected in humans, optimum conditions for short-chain polyglutamates (MTXPG1-3) were given priority. Consequently, the 1-cm window was chosen for analysis.

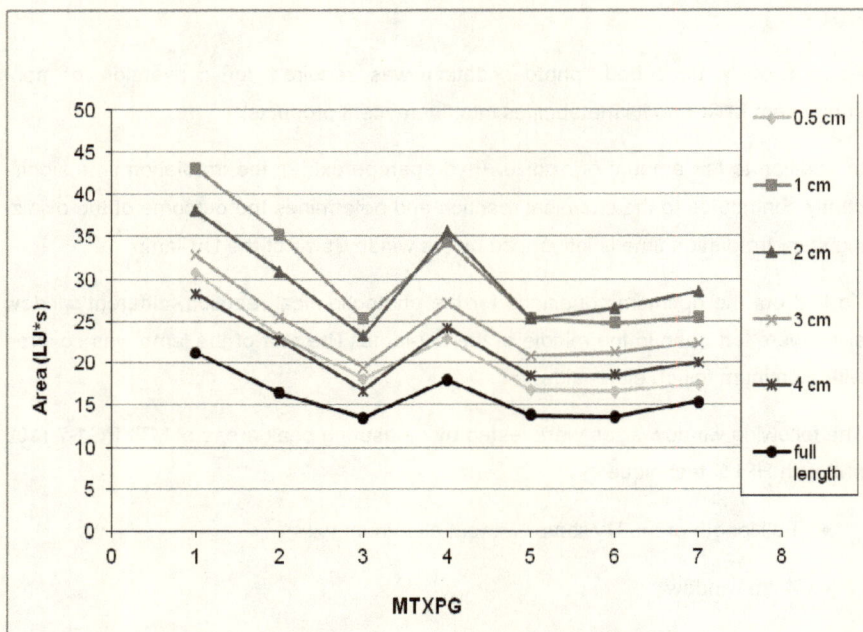

Figure 34: Peak Areas of MTXPG1-7 (100 nM) depending on UV-lamp-window-sizes left open

b) Co-Chromatography of MTXPG4 and MTXPG5

As already mentioned, interferences were observed at the chromatographic positions of MTXPG4 and MTXPG5 in blank patient's samples.

To ensure peak identity, co-chromatography of MTXPG4 and MTXPG5 was per-formed.

For that purpose, predefined amounts (100 nM) of MTXPG4 and MTXPG5 standard solutions were added to a patient's blank RBC sample.

The increase in peak areas assured that the interferences observed were identical with MTXPG4 and MTXPG5. Overlaid chromatograms of blank samples (black line) and co-chromatography (red line) are illustrated in figure 35.

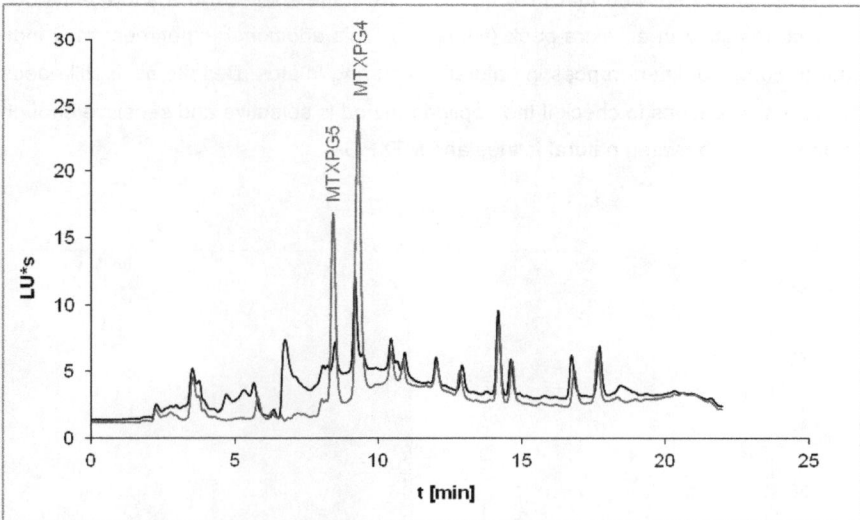

Figure 35: Co-Chromatography of MTXPG4 and MTXPG5 (red line) added to a patient's blank erythrocyte sample (black line) (overlaid chromatograms)

c) Hydrolysis of MTXPG4 and MTXPG5 using plasma

The result of co-chromatography raised the question, if PG4 and PG5 may occur as natural folates in erythrocytes. To clarify this question, PG4 and PG5 were hydrolyzed using blank plasma which naturally contains GGH (gamma-glutamyl hydrolase), an enzyme catalyzing the removal of polyglutamate tails.

In doing so, 50 µl patient´s RBC sample were homogenized with 50 µl of human blank plasma. For activation of GGH, probes were incubated for 1 hour at 37°C. Chromatography showed that PG4 and PG5 were metabolized to a shorter-chained product, resulting in an extra-peak (figure 36). This additional experiment may indicate the origin of interferences in naturally occurring folates. Despite all, it still needs further investigations to check if the applied method is selective and sensitive enough to differentiate between natural folates and MTXPGs.

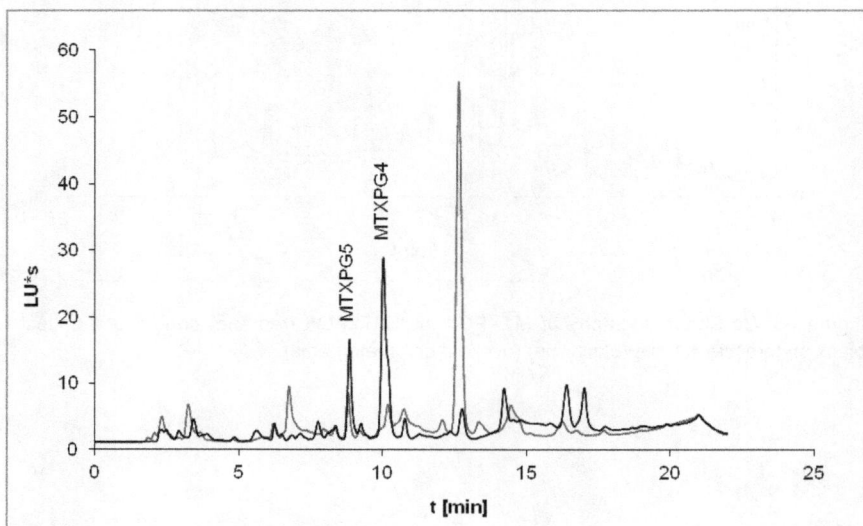

Figure 36: Hydrolysis of MTXPG4 and MTXPG5 using plasma; black line: before hydrolysis, red line: after hydrolysis using plasma-GGH (overlaid chromatograms)

3.4 DISCUSSION

After the optimization of two previously published HPLC methods [39, 77], plasma MTX and 7-hydroxymethotrexate as well as erythrocyte polyglutamates were analyzed. The distribution of MTX between plasma and erythrocytes – two different pharmacokinetic compartments – could be described by the combined use of these approaches.

Due to the fact that the major part of plasma MTX is excreted by the kidneys within the first 12 hours after administration, the importance of erythrocyte polyglutamates in drug monitoring was confirmed.

In erythrocytes, MTXPG1 occurred within 1.5 hours after drug administration. Interestingly, a redistribution of MTXPG1 to plasma MTX was observed 168 hours after MTX intake. Even though serum MTX was totally excreted by the kidneys within 48 hours, MTX recurred in this compartment shortly before the next administration. This phenomenon may be explained by a saturation mechanism of erythrocytes.

In general, formation of MTXPG2 and MTXPG3 started within 168 hours after MTX intake.

Steady-state of MTXPG1-3 was not achieved before week 10.

At this point it is necessary to mention that the extremly long accumulation half-lives of MTXPG1-3 (up to 46 weeks) should be unexceptionally understood as virtual values, which are in accordance with Dalrymple and co-workers [79]. The results of half-life calculation can not be explained by the physiological erythrocyte life duration of 120 days, but are relativized by the fact that lymphocytes and not erythrocytes are the actual target of methotrexate in the therapy of inflammatory diseases such as rheumatoid arthritis.

Nevertheless, concentrations of methotrexate polyglutamates were shown to correlate with clinical parameters and therefore may serve as marker for clinical response.

At week 5, C_{max} of *MTXPG1* negatively correlated with monocytes, which emphasizes the importance of polyglutamate accumulation in erythrocytes.

Monocytes are produced by the bone marrow from monoblasts and are a major part of the human immune system. Migration of peripheral blood mononuclear cells to inflamed synovium is the result of a cascade that involves several adhesion molecules. Infiltration of the synovium by monocytes is one of the main features in rheumatoid arthritis [80].

Supplemental to existing theories, *MTXPG2* was identified as a potential marker for clinical outcome in rheumatoid arthritis. There was a statistically significant positive correlation of MTXPG2 concentration and improvement in DAS-28. Higher levels of MTXPG2 went along with a significant reduction in DAS-28 at the end of the clinical trial at week 16. DAS-28 calculation incorporates clinical parameters (ESR, swollen and tender joints) as well as subjective parameters (VAS pain). Therefore, this correlation indicates the importance of MTXPG2 in drug monitoring. Up to now, only the accumulation of long-chained polyglutamates was linked to a good MTX response.

At week 5, a negative correlation between C_{max} levels of MTXPG2 and eosinophils was observed. Additionally, at week 10 even a negative correlation with basophils. Eosinophils and basophils are differentiating from myeloid precursor cells in response to interleukin-3, interleukin-5 and GM-CSF. Because eosinophils play a role in fibrin removal, eosinophilia is a typical characteristic for inflammation and rheumatoid arthritis. Further, increased circulating basophils are associated with rheumatic disorders, among them juvenile rheumatoid arthritis.

In contrast to MTXPG2, higher levels of *MTXPG3* seem to have a negative impact on disease improvement. This is particularly evident through a statistically significant positive correlation between C_{max} levels of MTXPG3 levels and ESR as well as CRP at week 5.

Explaining the pharmacokinetic profile of MTX, formation of polyglutamates in erythrocytes negatively correlated with C_{max} levels of MTX in plasma. Further, a positive correlation between C_{max} levels of MTX and 7-OH-MTX is evident.

Potential limits of the pharmacokinetic analysis were interferences at the chromatographic positions of MTXPG4 and MTXPG5. As a consequence, these polyglutamates were not included in data analysis.

By co-chromatography, interferences were identified as PG4 and PG5. By the use of hydrolysis, PG4 and PG5 were metabolized to a shorter-chained polyglutamate, resulting in an extra peak. This experiment may prove the natural occurrence of PG4 and PG5 in humans and subsequently relativizes the importance as potential outcome parameters in rheumatoid arthritis. For verification of these results, further investigations are needed.

Of clinical importance is the large inter- and intrapatient variability of methotrexate. In some cases, subcutaneous administration of MTX resulted in higher MTX and polyglutamate levels. In contrast, other patients achieved higher concentrations after methotrexate given orally. As a consequence, subcutaneous administration of MTX was not of a statistically significant benefit in this group of rheumatoaid arthritis patients (Wilcoxon-test for paired samples).

To compare the pharmacokinetics of a higher starting dose and a standard dose, 10 patients received a starting dose of 15 mg per week. Dose was escalated every two weeks until 25 mg per week. The second group (9 patients) immediately started with 25 mg MTX, given orally once a week.

This resulted in statistically higher C_{max}-levels of MTX and MTXPG1 in patients receiving 25 mg MTX per week (Mann-Whitney-U-test for independent samples).

However, the difference in pharmacokinetics was not relevant for clinical response, because a higher starting dose of MTX did not accelerate clinical response as compared to a standard dose.

As a conclusion, the combined analysis of serum MTX and erythrocyte polyglutamates describes the distribution of the drug between two different pharmacokinetic compartments and gives information about the detailed pharmacokinetic profile of methotrexate in rheumatoid arthritis.

It is of particular interest and supplementary to existing results, that MTXPG2 – a short-chained erythrocyte polyglutamate – was identified as a potential marker for clinical response in rheumatoid arthritis, correlating positively with improvement in DAS-28 and inversely with circulating eosinophils and basophils.

4 PHARMACOGENOMICS

4.1 INTRODUCTION

The influence of pharmacological treatment with methotrexate on the immune response of patients with rheumatoid arthritis was evaluated by real-time polymerase chain reaction (RT-PCR).

4.1.1 REAL-TIME PCR

Developed in the 1990s and based on the original polymerase chain reaction (PCR), real-time PCR technique allows monitoring the amount of product formed during the course of reaction.

Before starting RT-PCR, reverse transcription (RT) is required to copy mRNA to cDNA, obtaining higher efficacy when primers are added. Because the greatest yield of RT product is usually obtained by using short random oligonucleotides to prime the RT reaction, random primers are preferred for RNA of lower quality or when the template is limiting (i.e. archival samples).

DNA amplification is measured during PCR in "real-time" by the use of fluorophores. The fluorescence of probes in the reaction is proportional to the amount of product formed. The use of fluorescence reporter probes significantly increases the specificity of reaction, because only DNA containing the probe sequence is detected. This results in a probe with a fluorescent reporter at one and a quencher of fluorescence at the other side.

Taq®-Polymerase - a thermostable enzyme named after the bacterium thermus aquaticus (taq) - breaks down the reporter-quencher proximity by the 5′ to 3′ exonuclease activity, resulting in an unquenched emission of fluorescence. After excitation, fluorescence can be detected using a laser.

The number of DNA molecules initially present in the sample is calculated by registration of the number of amplification cycles required to obtain a certain amount of DNA molecules, assuming a particular amplification efficacy.

Gene expression analysis includes a typical use of RT-PCR [81].

4.1.2   GENE EXPRESSION ANALYSIS

mRNA concentrations of FPGS (folylpolyglutamate synthetase), GGH (gamma-glutamyl hydrolase), TNF (tumor necrosis factor), IL (interleukin)-6, IL-12A, IL-17A and IL-18 were determined in PBMCs (peripheral blood mononuclear cells) from 17 patients prior to and during methotrexate therapy.

4.1.2.1   GGH and FPGS

Gamma-glutamyl hydrolase (GGH), a lysosomal and secreted glycoprotein, hydrolyzes the gamma-glutamyl tail of folylpolyglutamates. In normal tissues, maximum levels of GGH mRNA are found in liver and kidneys. The low-affinity enzyme has a cysteine at the active site, which is suggested to be responsible for hydrolysis by attacking the gamma-amide linkage [82]. Hydrolysis of polyglutamate tails makes folates and antifolates exportable out of the cell. In contrast, the enzyme FPGS enables the cell to retain folates by addition of glutamate chains [83] and is essential for folate homeostasis and survival of proliferating cells. As a result of enhanced retention, the intracellular concentration of folates and antifolates is increased. In mammalian cells, FPGS activity is distributed to both cytosolic and mitochondrial compartments [84].

93

4.1.2.2   TNF

Involved in systemic inflammation, the prototypic cytokine of the TNF family stimulates an acute phase reaction.

The 212-amino acid long type II transmembrane protein – arranged in stable homotrimers – is a soluble 17-kd protein and produced by macrophages, monocytes, B-cells, T-cells and fibroblasts. By proteolytic cleavage, TNF is released from a cell membrane-anchored precursor. TNF induces other pro-inflammatory cytokines such as IL-1, IL-6, IL-8 as well as GM-CSF. Further, TNF stimulates fibroblasts to express adhesion molecules and therefore promotes inflammation. A local increase of TNF causes heat, swelling, redness and pain – typical symptoms of rheumatoid arthritis [85].

4.1.2.3   Interleukins

Interleukins - a group of cytokines - are mainly synthesized by CD4+-T-helper lymphocytes, monocytes, macrophages and endothelial cells and have important functions in regulating the immune system. They promote the development and differentiation of T-, B-, and hematopoietic cells. The chronic autoimmune response, which is characteristic of rheumatoid arthritis, is mediated by CD4+ T-cells. It was shown, that Th1-cells produce pro-inflammatory cytokines such as IL-2, IFN-γ and IL-12, activate macrophages and mediate cellular immunity. In contrast, Th2-cells secrete anti-inflammatory cytokines such as IL-4, IL-5 and IL-10 and down-modulate macrophage activation.

Therefore, imbalances in Th1/Th2-cytokines are associated with the pathogenesis of autoimmune-diseases [86].

a) Interleukin-6

IL-6 – encoded by the IL-6 gene - is an important cytokine involved in the pathogenesis of rheumatoid arthritis. Therefore, severe rheumatoid arthritis is treated with anti-IL-6 monoclonal antibodies. IL-6 acts as pro- as well as anti-inflammatory cytokine. The pleiotropic cytokine is produced by T-cells, monocytes, macrophages and synovial fibroblasts and is amongst others responsible for activation of T-cells, induction of acute-phase response and proliferation of synovial fibroblasts. Further, IL-6 is involved in B-cell proliferation and antibody production [87].

b) Interleukin 12A

IL-12 is mainly produced by antigen-presenting cells and has an important role in immunoregulation. The cytokine with a molecular weight of 70 kd is composed of two covalently-linked subunits (p35 and p40). There is a homology of the sequence of the p35 chain to that of IL-6. Further, the sequence of the p40 chain is homologous to the extracellular domain of the IL-6 receptor α-chain. These facts explain some of the actions involved in the mechanism of rheumatoid arthritis. Like IL-6, both subunits of the membrane receptor complex (IL-12R β1 and IL-12R β2) are members of class I cytokine receptor family [88]. IL-12 is produced by macrophages and dendritic cells in response to antigenic stimulation. The cytokine is involved in Th1-cell proliferation and maturation, T-cell and NK-cell cytotoxicity as well as B-cell activation [87].

c) Interleukin 17A

IL-17A, a pro-inflammatory Th1-cytokine, is produced by activated T-cells and plays an essential role in perpetuation of joint inflammation in rheumatoid arthritis. IL-17A is a 155-amino acid disulfide-linked homodimeric glycoprotein with a molecular weight of 35 kd. The IL-17 receptor (IL-17R) is a type I transmembrane protein consisting of a 293-amino acid extracellular domain, a 21-amino acid transmembrane domain and a 525-amino acid cytoplasmic tail [89].

IL-17 cooperates with IL-1β and TNF-α to promote inflammatory reactions [90] and enhances the production of IL-6 and IL-8 in synovial fibroblasts via activation of phosphatidylinositol 3-kinase/Akt and NF-κB [91].

d) Interleukin 18

IL-18, a member of IL-1 cytokine superfamily, is expressed at sites of chronic inflammation and is amongst others found in macrophages, dendritic cells, Kupffer cells, keratinocytes, osteoblasts and synovial fibroblasts. Pro-IL-18, an inactive precursor with a molecular weight of 24 kd, is converted to the biologically active 18-kd moiety either by the endoprotease IL-1ß converting enzyme (caspase-1) or by proteinase-3.

The heterodimer receptor complex (IL-18R) consists of an α-chain responsible for extracellular binding of IL-18 and a nonbinding ß-chain, which is required for signal transduction. Interaction with IL-12 results in an up-regulation of IL-18R on naive T-cells, Th1-cells and B-cells, whereas IL-4 implicates a down-regulation of the receptor complex.

Functionally, IL-18 induces T- and NK-cell maturation, cytokine production (TNF-α, GM-CSF, IFN-γ, IL-6) as well as cytotoxicity. Further, intracellular adhesion molecules such as ICAM-1 and VCAM-1 are up-regulated on endothelial cells and synovial fibroblasts. In the context of articular inflammation, these effects result in a pro-inflammatory effect of IL-18 [92, 93].

4.2 MATERIALS AND METHODS

4.2.1 REAGENTS AND MATERIALS

Tri Reagent® and mineral oil were obtained from Sigma (Saint Louis, USA). Chloroform, isopropanol and ethanol were bought from Merck (Darmstadt, Germany). HotStar Taq® DNA Polymerase, RNase Inhibitor, Q-solution and dNTP Mix were purchased from Qiagen (Vienna, Austria). Random primers were bought from Invitrogen (Lofer, Austria). Multiscribe Reverse Transcription TaqMan® Kit, TaqMan® Universal PCR Master Mix No AmpErase® UNG, Human GAPDH Endogenous Control, TaqMan® Ribosomal RNA Control Reagents, Hs00174128_m1 (TNF), Hs00909424_g1 (FPGS), Hs00914163_m1 (GGH), Hs99999032_m1 (IL-6), Hs00168405_m1 (IL-12A), Hs00174383_m1 (IL-17A), Hs99999040_m1 (IL-18), MicroAmp® Optical 96-well Reaction Plate with Barcode and MicroAmp® Optical 8-Cap Strips were obtained from Applied Biosystems (Vienna, Austria). ß-Actin primer (3/P, 4/M) were bought from VBC Biotech (Vienna, Austria). Biocoll® solution and PBS-solution were purchased from Biochrom AG (Berlin, Germany). RNase-free water (DEPC water) was used.

4.2.2   RNA PREPARATION

As previously described for preparation of plasma and RBCs, EDTA-whole blood (6 ml) was drawn from rheumatoid arthritis patients and stored up to four hours at 4°C until further processing. For gene expression analysis, the following blood samples were edited:

- Pre-value before starting MTX therapy

- Pre-value week 5

- 4-hour-value week 5

- Pre-value week 6

6 ml of Biocoll® solution were laid in a 15 ml conical tube before carefully adding 6 ml of EDTA-blood, using a pipette.

After a 20-min centrifugation step (1600 RPM, 4°C) to separate plasma and RBCs from buffy coat (leukocytes and platelets), leukocytes were washed twice with 14 ml PBS-solution and centrifuged for 10 min at 1000 RPM (4°C).

After counting cells, leukocytes were lysed in Tri Reagent® by repeated pipeting. Tri Reagent® is a mixture of guanidine thiocyanate and phenol in a mono-phase solution, which effectively dissolves DNA, RNA and protein. One ml of reagent is sufficient to lyse 5-10 x10^6 cells. Therefore, on average 1.5 ml of reagent were needed per patient sample. After homogenization and a 5-min incubation step, samples were stored at -80°C for up to 1 month. After thawing, 0.2 ml of chloroform per ml Tri Reagent® was added. Next, samples were vortexed for 15 seconds and incubated for 15 minutes at room temperature. Centrifugation at 8000 RPM for 15 minutes at 4°C separated the mixture into 3 phases:

- Protein phase (red organic phase)

- DNA phase (interphase)

- RNA phase (colorless upper aqueous phase)

The aqueous phase was transferred into a fresh tube before adding 0.5 ml of isopropanol per ml Tri Reagent®. After repeated pipeting, the mixture was incubated for 10 minutes at room temperature. After centrifugation at 8000 RPM for 10 minutes at 4°C, the RNA precipitate formed a pellet on side walls and on the bottom of the tube.

The supernatant was removed and the RNA pellet was washed with 1 ml of 75% ethanol per 1 ml Tri Reagent®. After vortexing and centrifugation at 6000 RPM for 5 min at 4°C, the RNA pellet was dried for 10 minutes by air-drying. Finally, 20 μl of DEPC-water was added before performing spectrophotometry to check quality and quantity of RNA.

For spectrophotometry, 1 μl of RNA sample was diluted with 69 μl of 0.9% sodium chloride (1:70 dilution) and measured using a ratio of E260 nm/E280 nm. A ratio of E260/E280 around 2 indicates good RNA quality.

For calculation of RNA concentration, the following formula was applied. The multiplication factor of 40 is used to incorporate the hyperchromatic effect of RNA:

$$E(260\ nm) \times 40 \times 70 = \mu g\ \frac{RNA}{ml}$$

$$\mu g\ \frac{RNA/ml}{1000} = \mu g\ \frac{RNA}{\mu l}$$

$$\mu g\ RNA/\mu l \times 20 = \mu g\ RNA\ in\ 20\ \mu l$$

For quality control of RNA, *gel electrophoresis* was carried out. Gel electrophoresis is a technique to separate for example RNA using an electric field, applied to a gel matrix. Therefore an agarose gel (1% agarose in TBE puffer, 1x) was made. Agarose is composed of long unbranched chains of uncharged carbohydrate without cross links, resulting in a gel with large pores. This circumstance allows the separation of macromolecules.

99

Before starting, the gel chamber was cleaned using RNase ERASE® to remove RNase contamination. The used RNA concentration was 1 μg in a total volume of 10 μl. For that purpose, the calculated amount of RNA was mixed with DEPC-water and filled up to a total volume of 10 μl. Additionally, 10 μl of denaturation puffer was added to each vial. After a 3-minute heating step using a gradient block at 65°C, probes were cooled on ice for 5 minutes. Finally, samples were centrifuged for 30 seconds at 6000 RPM and loaded onto the gel.

Gel electrophoresis was performed at 80 Volt for 3 hours.

In figure 37, a photograph of a gel, taken under ultraviolet lighting conditions and showing patient's RNA samples, is presented. The three different RNA bands (28S-RNA, 18S-RNA and transfer RNA) are clearly visible and indicate intact RNA samples.

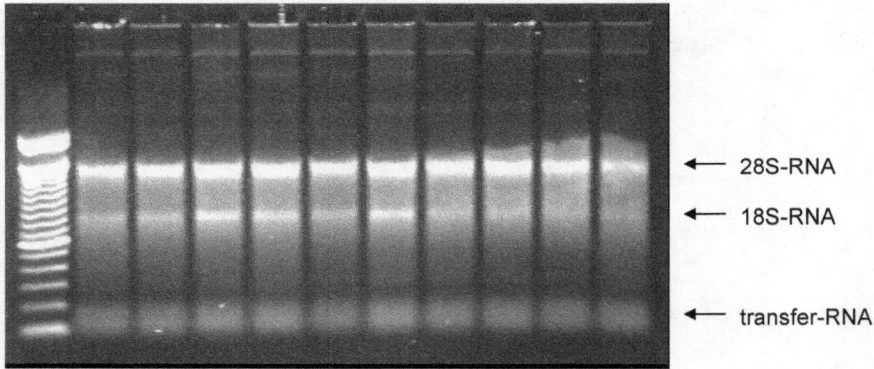

Figure 37: Photograph of a gel showing patient's RNA samples (far left: DNA marker)

4.2.3   CDNA SYNTHESIS

Catalyzed by the enzyme reverse transcriptase, cDNA (complementary DNA) was synthesized from a mature mRNA template using random primers and dNTPs (dGTP, dCTP, dATP, dTTP) (figure 38). cDNA is much more stable than RNA, which is easily degraded by RNases.

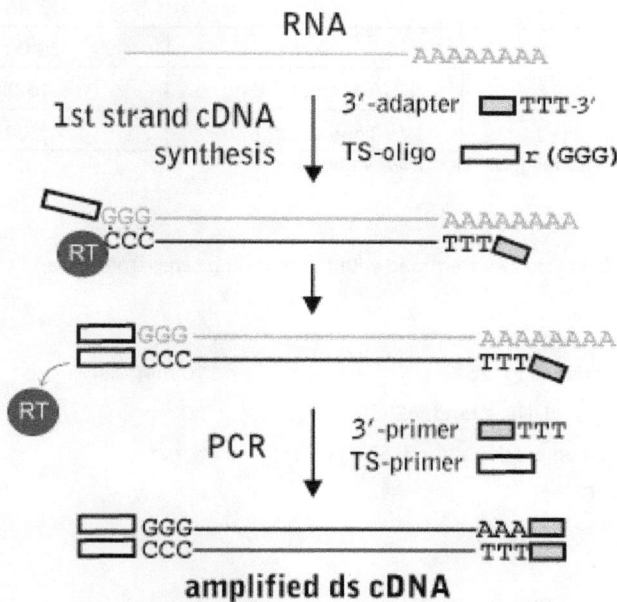

Figure 38: Synthesis of the first strand of cDNA using a primer and reverse transcriptase (http://evrogen.ru/technologies/SMART.shtml, last checked 17/06/2010)

The following reagents were needed for cDNA synthesis:

Reagents	Concentration	µl/sample
dNTPs	100 mM	0.45 µl
Multiscribe RT-Puffer	10x	4.50 µl
Multiscribe RT	50 U/µl	3.00 µl
RNase Inhibitor	20 U/µl	0.57 µl
Random primer	0.3 µg/µl	3.00 µl
DEPC water	-	18.48 µl
	Volume	30.00 µl
	RNA 2 ng/µl (30 ng)	+ 15.00 µl
	Total volume	45.00 µl

Table 13: Required reagents for cDNA synthesis

The thermocycler was programmed with the following temperatures and times:

- Primer annealing: 25°C   10 min
- Forming of cDNA strand: 42°C   30 min   } 1x
- Degradation of RNA strand: 85°C   5 min
- Hold: 4°C

To check cDNA synthesis, PCR (polymerase chain reaction) was performed for amplification of the ß-actin gene (housekeeping gene). For that purpose, thin-walled PCR tubes and the following reagents were used:

Reagents	Concentration	µl/sample
PCR-puffer + MgCl$_2$	10x	5.0 µl
Q1-solution	5x	10.0 µl
dNTP-mix	2 mM	5.0 µl
ß-actin 3/P	5 µM	2.5 µl
ß-actin 4/M	5 µM	2.5 µl
DEPC water	-	22.5 µl
Hot Star Taq™DNA-polymerase	5 U/µl	0.5 µl
	Volume	48.0 µl
	cDNA (0.667 ng/µl)	+ 2.0 µl
	Total volume	50.0 µl

Table 14: Required reagents for PCR (amplification of the ß-actin gene)

The total volume was overlaid with 50 µl of mineral oil before starting PCR with the following thermocycler program:

- Denaturation: 95°C   15 min
- Primer annealing: 60°C   1 min   } 1x
- Amplification: 72°C   1 min

- Denaturation: 95°C   1 min
- Primer annealing: 60°C   1 min   } 34x
- Amplification: 72°C   1 min

- Amplification: 72°C   10 min   } 1x
- Hold: 4°C

Finally, reaction products were analyzed by agarose gel electrophoresis (1% agarose gel in 1x TBE-puffer). 10 µl of the PCR product was mixed with 5 µl gel loading solution and loaded onto the gel.

The gel loading solution consisted of:

- 0.05% Orange gel
- 40% Sucrose
- 0.1 M EDTA
- 0.5% SDS (Sodium Dodecyl Sulfate)
- Aqua bidest.

Gel electrophoresis was performed at 180 Volt for 75 minutes. In figure 39, a photograph of a gel is presented. The bands of ß-actin, the housekeeping gene, are clearly visible and serve as a marker for quality control.

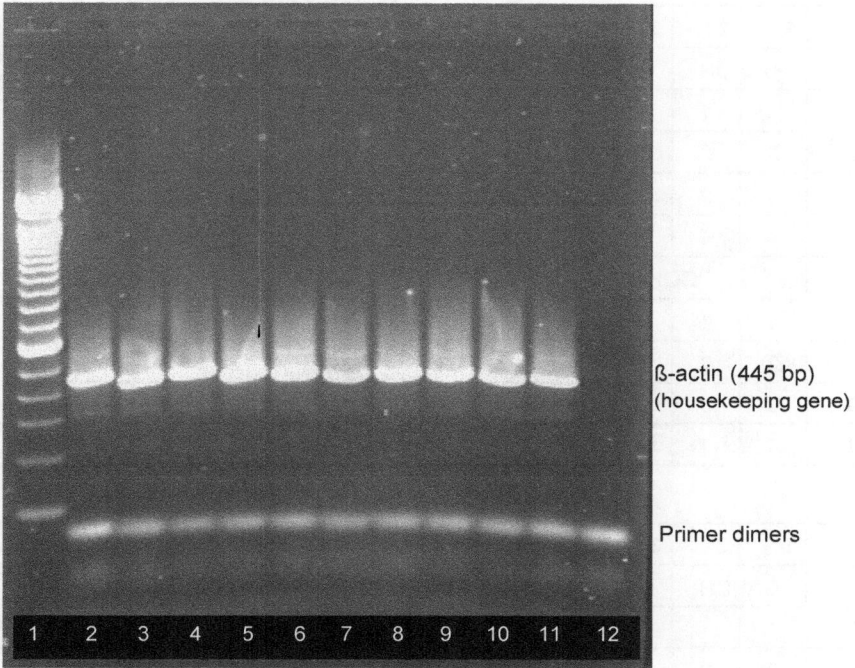

Figure 39: Photograph of a gel showing amplification of cDNA

1. 100 bp DNA marker (0.5 µg)
2.-11. Amplificat of 2 µl cDNA (patient samples)
12. Blank sample (reagent control)

4.2.4 REAL-TIME PCR

To quantify differences in mRNA expression of seven different genes (FPGS, GGH, TNF, IL-6, IL-12A, IL-17A and IL-18), real-time PCR was performed. GAPDH was used as endogenous control. For each patient, two 96-well reaction plates were designed (figure 40). Each value was repeated four times.

	1	2	3	4	5	6	7	8	9	10	11	12
	GAPDH		18-S-RNA		TNF				FPGS			
A	1	1	1	1	1	1	1	1	1	1	1	1
B	2	2	2	2	2	2	2	2	2	2	2	2
C	3	3	3	3	3	3	3	3	3	3	3	3
D	4	4	4	4	4	4	4	4	4	4	4	4
	GGH				IL-6				Negative control			
E	1	1	1	1	1	1	1	1	1	1	1	1
F	2	2	2	2	2	2	2	2	2	2	2	2
G	3	3	3	3	3	3	3	3	3	3	3	3
H	4	4	4	4	4	4	4	4	4	4	4	4

	1	2	3	4	5	6	7	8	9	10	11	12
	GAPDH		18-S-RNA		IL-12A				IL-17A			
A	1	1	1	1	1	1	1	1	1	1	1	1
B	2	2	2	2	2	2	2	2	2	2	2	2
C	3	3	3	3	3	3	3	3	3	3	3	3
D	4	4	4	4	4	4	4	4	4	4	4	4
	IL-18				Negative control							
E	1	1	1	1	1	1	1	1				
F	2	2	2	2	2	2	2	2				
G	3	3	3	3	3	3	3	3				
H	4	4	4	4	4	4	4	4				

Figure 40: Design of 96-well reaction plates for one patient (1: Week 1 – pre-value, 2: Week 5 – pre-value, 3: Week 5 – 4 hours, 4: Week 6 – pre-value)

A master mix, containing TaqMan® Universal PCR Master Mix, DEPC water and TaqMan® probes, was prepared (table 15). 1.33 µl of cDNA sample was placed in each well before adding 22.67 µl of master mix. MicroAmp® Optical 8-Cap Strips were used to close plates before centrifugation at 1500 RPM for 3 minutes at ambient temperature.

Reagents	Concentration	µl/well
TaqMan® Universal PCR Master Mix	2x	12.00 µl
DEPC water	-	10.17 µl
TaqMan® probe	20x	0.50 µl
	Volume	22.67 µl
	cDNA	+ 1.33 µl
	Total volume	24.00 µl

Table 15: Required reagents for real-time PCR

For amplification, the ABI Prism 7700 Sequence Detection System was programmed with the following times and temperatures:

- Denaturation, Activation of AmpliTaq®-Gold: 95°C   10 min   } 1x
- Denaturation: 95°C   15 sec   } 50x
- Primer annealing, Amplification: 60°C   60 sec

4.3 RESULTS

Overall, 17 patients of the study population agreed to participate in gene expression studies.

Relative mRNA gene expression in PBMCs was analyzed using the Δ Ct method. The $2^{-\Delta\Delta Ct}$ method was used to calculate relative changes in gene expression. For this experiment, the pre-value sample drawn at week 1 before starting MTX therapy was selected as calibrator.

$$\Delta \ Ct = Ct \ (target) - Ct \ (endogenous \ control, \ GAPDH)$$
$$\Delta\Delta \ Ct = \Delta \ Ct \ (sample) - \Delta \ Ct \ (calibrator)$$

Statistically significant changes in mRNA gene expression were observed for TNF, FPGS, IL-6, IL12-A and IL-18.

IL-17A was not expressed on mRNA level in PBMCs and therefore not analyzed in detail. Although some alterations in GGH gene expression were noted, these were not of significance (see table 16).

4.3.1   DESCRIPTIVE STATISTICS

Table 16 presents the results of descriptive statistics including minimum, maximum and mean levels of relative gene expression (Δ Ct method).

As mentioned above, four different samples of each patient (week 1 pre-values, week 5 pre-values, week 5 4-hour values, week 6 pre-values) were analyzed.

Parameter	Mean (± SD)	Minimum	Maximum
FPGS			
Week 1 Pre-value	5.89 (± 0.85)	4.42	7.19
Week 5 Pre-value	6.15 (± 0.85)	4.91	7.76
Week 5 4 hours	6.15 (± 0.76)	4.60	7.31
Week 6 Pre-value	6.49 (± 0.90)	5.13	7.93
GGH			
Week 1 Pre-value	9.43 (± 0.77)	8.13	10.77
Week 5 Pre-value	9.54 (± 0.68)	8.45	10.63
Week 5 4 hours	9.48 (± 0.95)	8.02	11.25
Week 6 Pre-value	9.87 (± 0.72)	8.29	11.16
TNF			
Week 1 Pre-value	6.91 (± 0.74)	5.59	8.06
Week 5 Pre-value	7.16 (± 0.74)	6.02	8.68
Week 5 4 hours	6.87 (± 0.66)	5.53	7.69
Week 6 Pre-value	7.13 (± 0.73)	5.57	8.56
IL-6			
Week 1 Pre-value	19.91 (± 7.36)	11.00	28.60
Week 5 Pre-value	24.23 (± 6.02)	12.54	29.90
Week 5 4 hours	24.66 (± 5.76)	11.77	28.60
Week 6 Pre-value	24.50 (± 5.59)	13.22	28.79
IL-12A			
Week 1 Pre-value	11.28 (± 1.11)	9.16	13.02
Week 5 Pre-value	11.92 (± 0.91)	9.87	13.13
Week 5 4 hours	11.72 (± 1.05)	9.69	13.55
Week 6 Pre-value	11.98 (± 0.93)	10.16	13.56

Table 16a: Descriptive statistics of real-time PCR parameters using the Δ Ct method (endogenous control: GAPDH)

Parameter	Mean (± SD)	Minimum	Maximum
IL-17A			
Week 1 Pre-value	27.76 (± 0.75)	26.66	29.01
Week 5 Pre-value	27.47 (± 1.12)	25.15	29.87
Week 5 4 hours	27.33 (± 0.79)	25.81	28.61
Week 6 Pre-value	27.60 (± 0.71)	26.56	28.65
IL-18			
Week 1 Pre-value	9.42 (± 0.90)	7.35	10.99
Week 5 Pre-value	9.61 (± 0.92)	7.79	11.64
Week 5 4 hours	9.78 (± 0.85)	7.88	11.22
Week 6 Pre-value	9.81 (± 0.95)	7.74	11.98

Table 16b: Descriptive statistics of real-time PCR parameters using the Δ Ct method (endogenous control: GAPDH)

Using the $2^{-\Delta\Delta Ct}$ method, relative changes in gene expression were calculated. Results of descriptive statistics are presented in table 17. The pre-value sample taken before starting MTX therapy was used as calibrator.

Due to a large inter-patient variability, results are not well-defined. Hence, there is just a recognizable trend towards changes in the gene expression of FPGS, IL-6, IL-12A and IL-18.

Parameter	Mean (± SD)	Minimum	Maximum
FPGS			
Week 5 Pre-value	0.89 (± 0.32)	0.40	1.68
Week 5 4 hours	0.87 (± 0.25)	0.42	1.37
Week 6 Pre-value	0.70 (± 0.24)	0.31	1.36
GGH			
Week 5 Pre-value	0.99 (± 0.38)	0.38	2.00
Week 5 4 hours	1.18 (± 1.00)	0.48	4.58
Week 6 Pre-value	0.85 (± 0.52)	0.24	2.58
TNF			
Week 5 Pre-value	0.91 (± 0.33)	0.29	1.37
Week 5 4 hours	1.09 (± 0.44)	0.59	2.39
Week 6 Pre-value	0.97 (± 0.49)	0.32	2.00
IL-6			
Week 5 Pre-value	0.37 (± 0.63)	0.00	1.91
Week 5 4 hours	0.36 (± 0.64)	0.00	1.88
Week 6 Pre-value	0.17 (± 0.23)	0.00	0.60
IL-12A			
Week 5 Pre-value	0.69 (± 0.29)	0.39	1.51
Week 5 4 hours	0.85 (± 0.53)	0.29	2.21
Week 6 Pre-value	0.71 (± 0.40)	0.23	1.63
IL-18			
Week 5 Pre-value	0.92 (± 0.26)	0.42	1.29
Week 5 4 hours	0.85 (± 0.38)	0.31	1.92
Week 6 Pre-value	0.81 (± 0.29)	0.37	1.48

Table 17: Descriptive statistics of real-time PCR parameters presenting relative changes in gene expression using the $2^{-\Delta\Delta Ct}$ method

4.3.2 CORRELATION OF CYTOKINE GENE EXPRESSION AND PHARMACOKINETICS

Statistically significant correlations using the Spearman´s correlation coefficient are shown in table 18.

At week 5, a negative correlation of erythrocyte MTXPG1 C_{max} levels and TNF, IL-6 as well as IL-12A was found – implicating that higher C_{max} levels of MTXPG1 correlate with lower levels of pro-inflammatory cytokines (presented in table 18).

Interestingly, erythrocyte AUC levels of MTXPG1 and MTXPG2 as well as erythrocyte C_{max} levels of MTXPG2 and MTXPG3 positively correlated with IL-18, meaning that a higher gene expression of IL-18 is linked to higher concentrations of MTXPG1 and MTXPG2 (table 18). These findings are in accordance to the publication of Moeller and co-workers, who described that the constitutive expression of IL-18 mRNA is significantly reduced in rheumatoid arthritis PBMCs [94]. The fact that IL-18 stimulates the production of IL-1ß and TNF in vitro and that IL-18 is enhanced in synovial tissues may be a possible explanation for this phenomenon.

All things considered, the presented results may provide evidence of MTX's positive impact on inflammatory conditions.

Parameter	Correlation partner	Correlation	Significance (two-sided)
TNF			
Week 5 Pre-value	MTXPG1 C_{max} (nM) Week 5	- 0.651	0.005**
Week 5 Mean	MTXPG1 C_{max} (nM) Week 5	- 0.500	0.041*
IL-6			
Week 5 Mean	MTXPG1 C_{max} (nM) Week 5	- 0.534	0.027*
IL-12A			
Week 5 Pre-value	MTXPG1 C_{max} (nM) Week 5	- 0.657	0.004**
Week 5 Mean	MTXPG1 C_{max} (nM) Week 5	- 0.549	0.022*
Week 5 4 hours	MTXPG3 T_{max} (h) Week 5	- 0.698	0.002**
Week 5 Mean	MTXPG3 T_{max} (h) Week 5	- 0.541	0.025*
IL-18			
Week 5 Pre-value	MTXPG1 AUC (nM*h) Week 5	+ 0.485	0.048*
Week 5 Pre-value	MTXPG2 AUC (nM*h) Week 5	+ 0.635	0.006**
Week 5 Pre-value	MTXPG2 C_{max} (nM) Week 5	+ 0.566	0.018*
Week 5 Pre-value	MTXPG3 C_{max} (nM) Week 5	+ 0.610	0.009**
Week 5 4 hours	MTXPG2 AUC (nM*h) Week 5	+ 0.574	0.016*
Week 5 Mean	MTXPG2 AUC (nM*h) Week 5	+ 0.607	0.010**

Table 18: Correlation analysis of cytokine gene expression and pharmacokinetic parameters using the Spearman's correlation coefficient

Figures 41-46 present selected scatter-plots, showing the correlations of TNF, IL-6, IL-12A and IL-18 with MTXPG1 as well as correlations of IL-18 with MTXPG2 and MTXPG3.

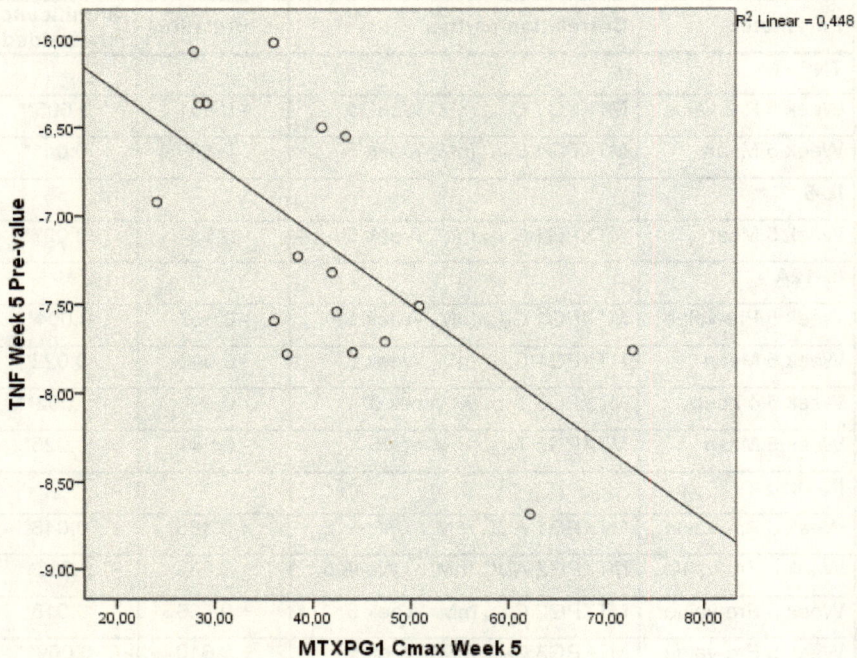

Figure 41: Scatter-plot: Correlation of MTXPG1 (C_{max}, nM) and gene expression of TNF (Week 5, Pre-value, Δ Ct)

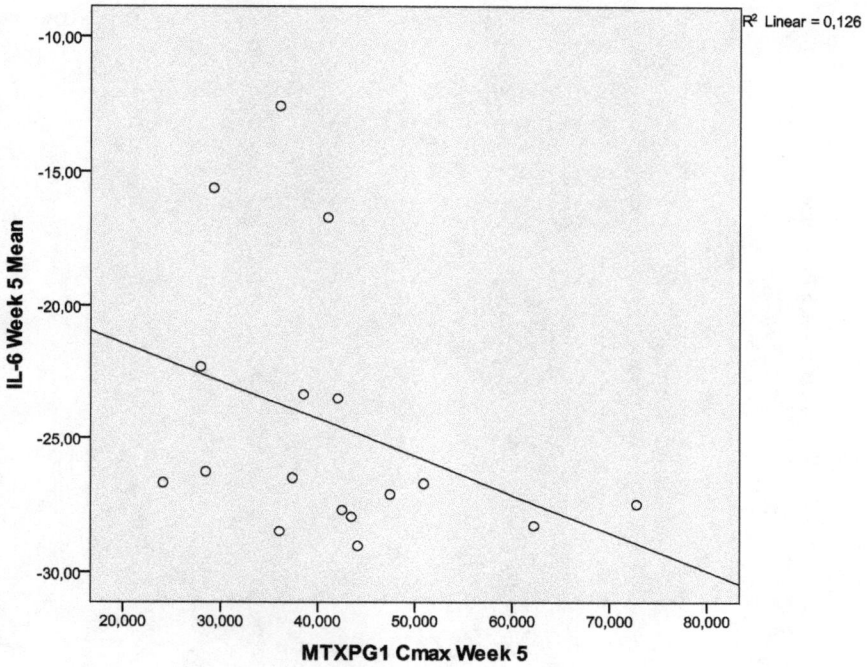

Figure 42: Scatter-plot: Correlation of MTXPG1 (C_{max}, nM) and gene expression of IL-6 (Week 5, Mean, Δ Ct)

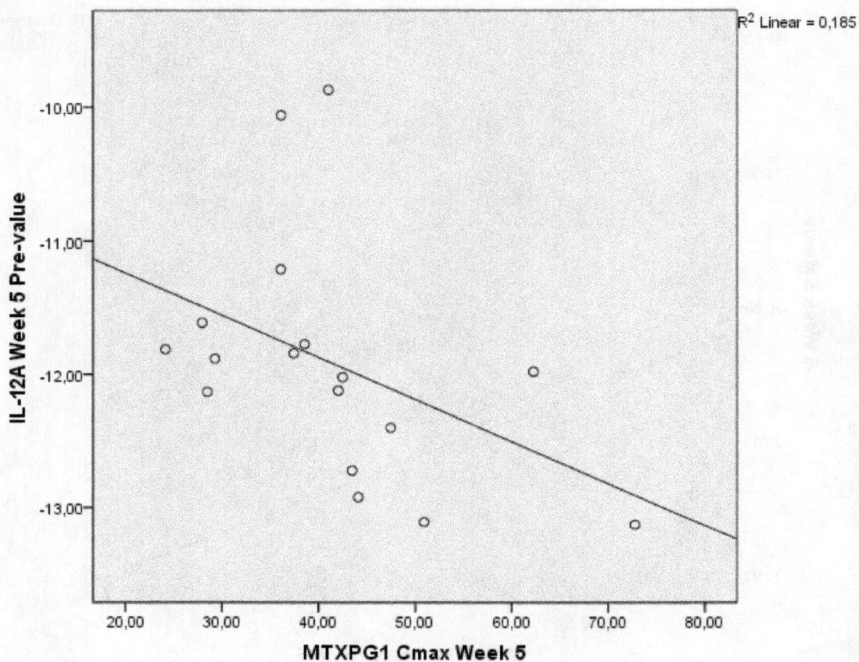

Figure 43: Scatter-plot: Correlation of MTXPG1 (C_{max}, nM) and gene expression of IL-12A (Week 5, Pre-value, Δ Ct)

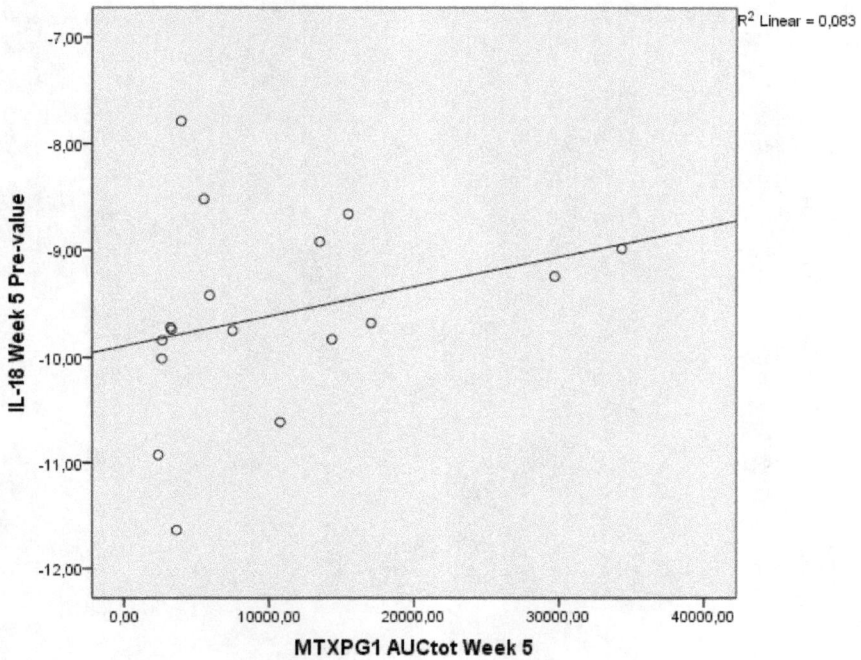

Figure 44: Scatter-plot: Correlation of MTXPG1 (AUC, nM*h) and gene expression of IL-18 (Week 5, Pre-value, Δ Ct)

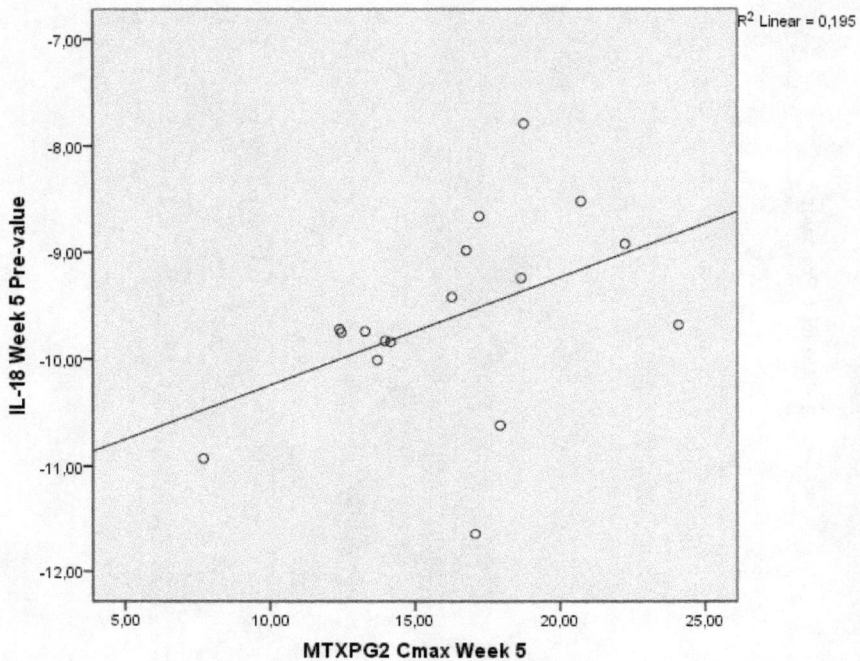

Figure 45: Scatter-plot: Correlation of MTXPG2 (C_{max}, nM) and gene expression of IL-18 (Week 5, Pre-value, Δ Ct)

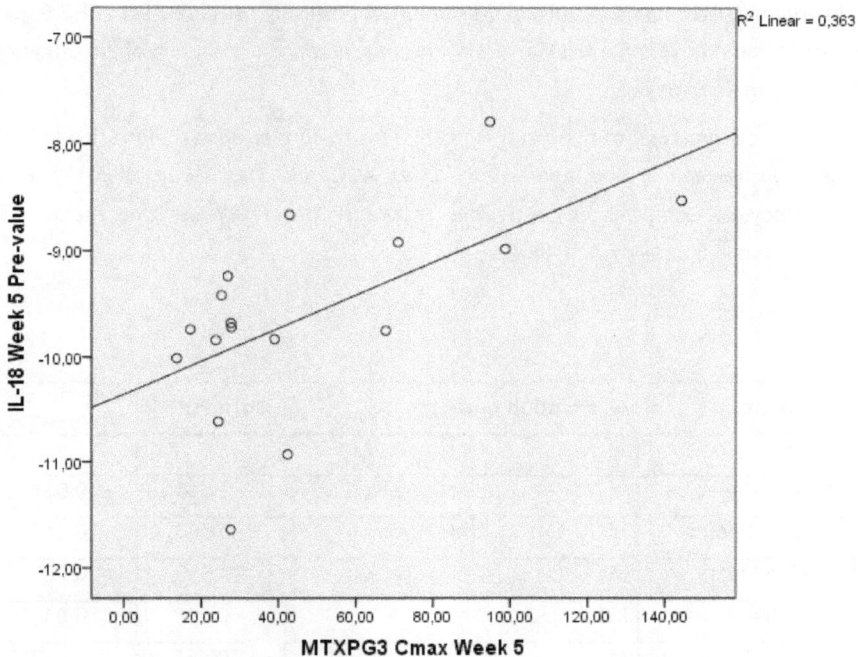

Figure 46: Scatter-plot: Correlation of MTXPG3 (C_{max}, nM) and gene expression of IL-18 (Week 5, Pre-value, Δ Ct)

4.3.3 CORRELATION OF FPGS AND GGH WITH PHARMACO-KINETIC PARAMETERS

A negative correlation of MTXPG1 erythrocyte C_{max} levels and mRNA expression of FPGS (4 hours value) was observed, showing that FPGS is a short acting enzyme with enhanced activity directly after methotrexate intake. The addition of gamma-glutamyl-chains and therefore FPGS activation comes along with reduced levels of MTXPG1.

In contrast, AUC and C_{max} levels of serum MTX positively correlated with FPGS gene expression 4 hours after MTX intake, which indicates the distribution of the drug from plasma to erythrocytes.

Due to low amounts of substrate for GGH, it was further shown that a lower GGH gene expression is accompanied by lower AUC and C_{max} levels of MTXPG2 in erythrocytes – presented by a positive correlation (table 19). Selected scatter-plots are shown in figures 47 and 48.

Parameter	Correlation partner	Correlation	Significance (two-sided)
FPGS			
Week 5 Pre-value	MTXPG1 C_{max} (nM) Week 5	- 0.510	0.037*
Week 5 4 hours	MTXPG1 C_{max} (nM) Week 5	- 0.586	0.013*
Week 5 Mean	MTXPG1 C_{max} (nM) Week 5	- 0.539	0.026*
Week 5 4 hours	MTX AUC (nM*h) Week 5	+ 0.598	0.011*
Week 5 Pre-value	MTX C_{max} (nM) Week 5	+ 0.485	0.048*
GGH			
Week 5 Mean	MTXPG2 AUC (nM*h) Week 5	+ 0.542	0.025*
Week 5 4 hours	MTXPG2 C_{max} (nM) Week 5	+ 0.483	0.050*
Week 5 Mean	MTXPG2 C_{max} (nM) Week 5	+ 0.589	0.013*
Week 5 Pre-value	MTX AUC (nM*h) Week 5	+ 0.522	0.032*

Table 19: Correlation analysis of FPGS and GGH gene expression and pharmacokinetic parameters using Spearman's correlation coefficient

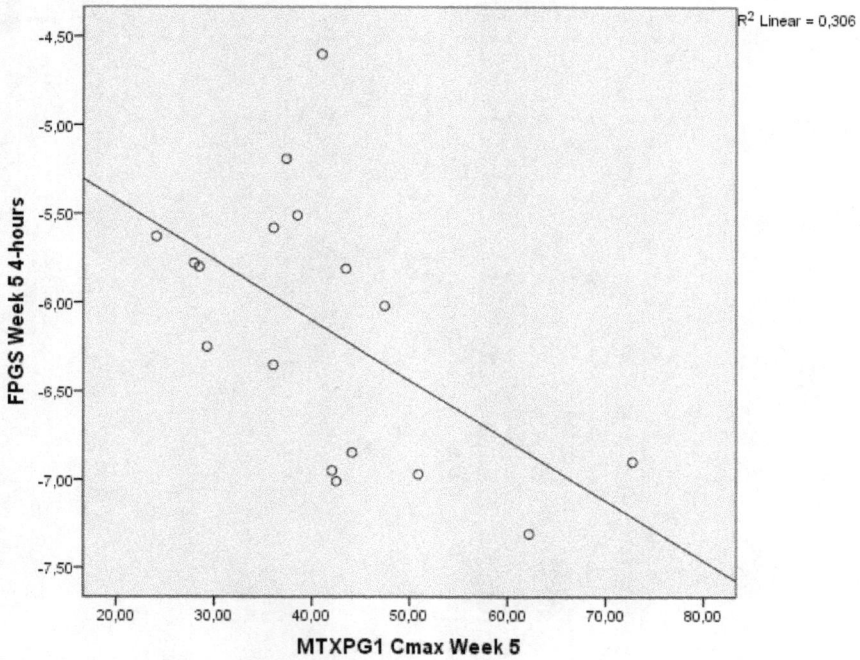

Figure 47: Scatter-plot: Correlation of MTXPG1 (C_{max}, nM) and gene expression of FPGS (Week 5, 4-hours-value, Δ Ct)

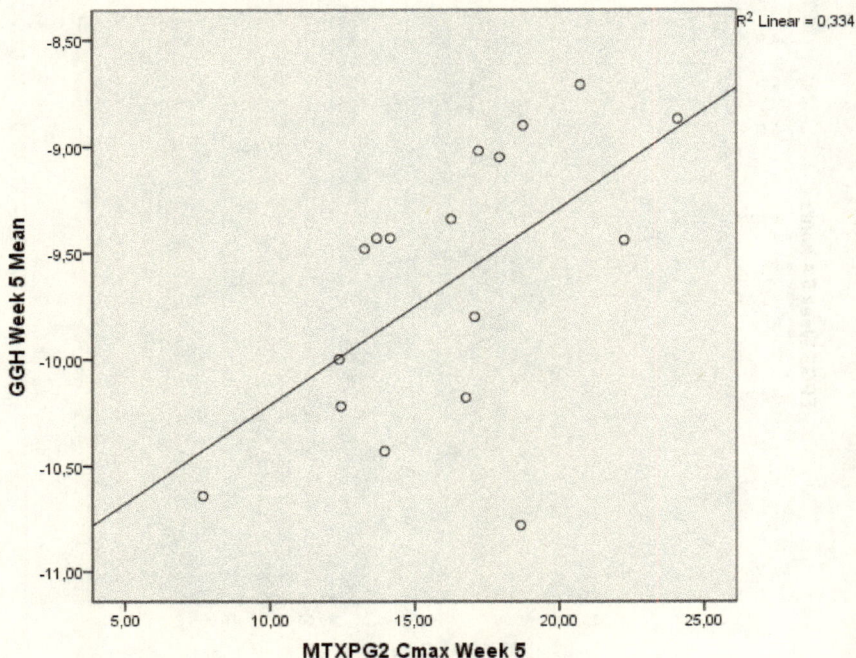

Figure 48: Scatter-plot: Correlation of MTXPG2 (C_{max}, nM) and gene expression of GGH (Week 5, Mean, Δ Ct)

4.3.4 CORRELATION OF CYTOKINE GENE EXPRESSION AND CLINICAL PARAMETERS

A positive correlation of TNF and monocytes was observed (p=0.040) after week 5, meaning that a depressed TNF gene expression is accompanied by lower levels of monocytes.

Gene expression of IL-12A positively correlated with CRP (p=0.005) and ANC (p=0.034), both important markers in rheumatology. Because IL-12A may be produced by basophils and eosinophils, a highly significant negative correlation with these markers is presented.

IL-18 was shown to have a high impact on inflammatory parameters, resulting in significant positive correlations of IL-18 gene expression with ESR (p=0.007), leukocytes, CRP and ANC at week 5. Therefore, a lower IL-18 gene expression involves a reduction in inflammatory parameters mentioned above. Results are presented in table 20.

Figures 49 to 52 present selected scatter-plots, showing the correlations of IL-12A with CRP and of IL-18 with CRP, leukocytes and ANC.

Parameter	Correlation partner	Correlation	Significance (two-sided)
TNF			
Week 5 Pre-value	Monocytes (%) Week 5	+ 0.503	0.040*
IL-12A			
Week 5 Pre-value	CRP (mg/l) Week 5	+ 0.647	0.005**
Week 5 4 hours	ANC (/nl) Week 5	+ 0.517	0.034*
Week 5 4 hours	Eosinophils (%) Week 5	- 0.647	0.005**
Week 5 Pre-value	Basophils (%) Week 5	- 0.541	0.025*
Week 5 4 hours	Basophils (%) Week 5	- 0.667	0.003**
Week 5 Mean	Basophils (%) Week 5	- 0.533	0.028*
IL-18			
Week 5 4 hours	ESR (mm/h) Week 5	+ 0.631	0.007**
Week 5 Pre-value	Leukocytes (/nl) Week 5	+ 0.645	0.005**
Week 5 4 hours	Leukocytes (/nl) Week 5	+ 0.642	0.005**
Week 5 Mean	Leukocytes (/nl) Week 5	+ 0.555	0.021*
Week 5 Pre-value	CRP (mg/l) Week 5	+ 0.669	0.003**
Week 5 Mean	CRP (mg/l) Week 5	+ 0.605	0.010*
Week 5 Pre-value	ANC (/nl) Week 5	+ 0.672	0.003**
Week 5 4 hours	ANC (/nl) Week 5	+ 0.555	0.021*
Week 5 Mean	ANC (/nl) Week 5	+ 0.519	0.033*

Table 20: Correlation analysis of cytokine gene expression and clinical parameters using the Spearman's correlation coefficient

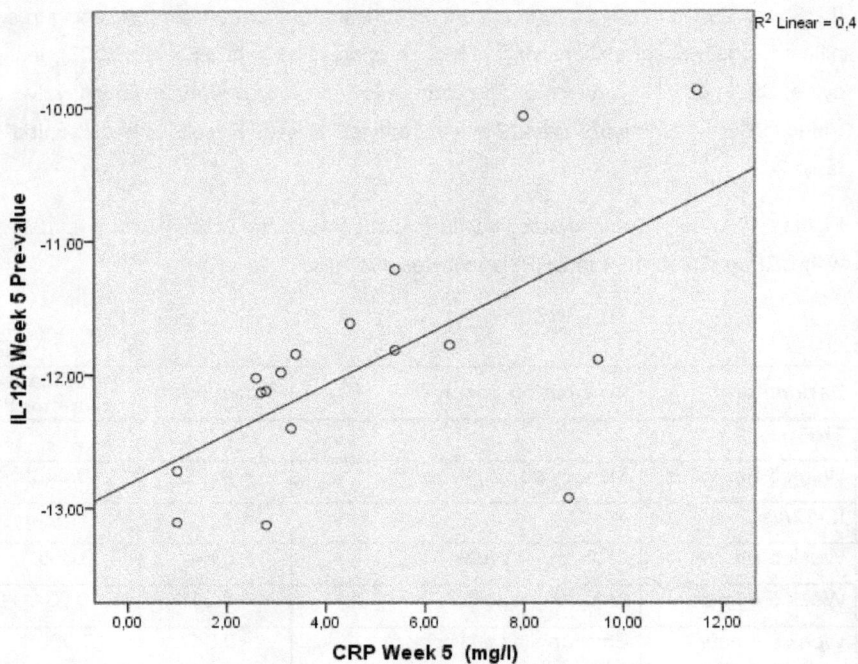

Figure 49: Scatter-plot: Correlation of CRP (Week 5, mg/l) and gene expression of IL-12A (Week 5, Pre-Value, Δ Ct)

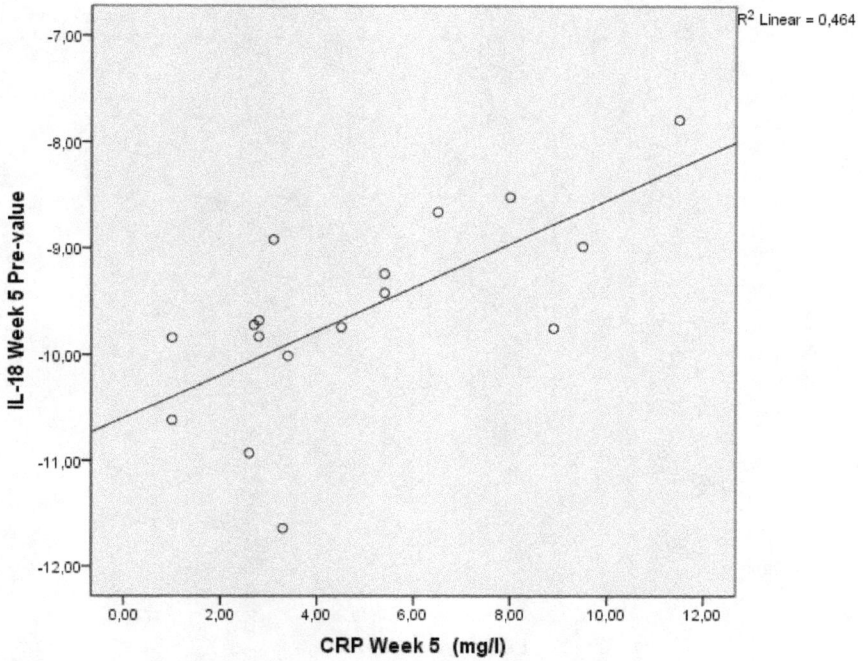

Figure 50: Scatter-plot: Correlation of CRP (Week 5, mg/l) and gene expression of IL-18 (Week 5, Pre-Value, Δ Ct)

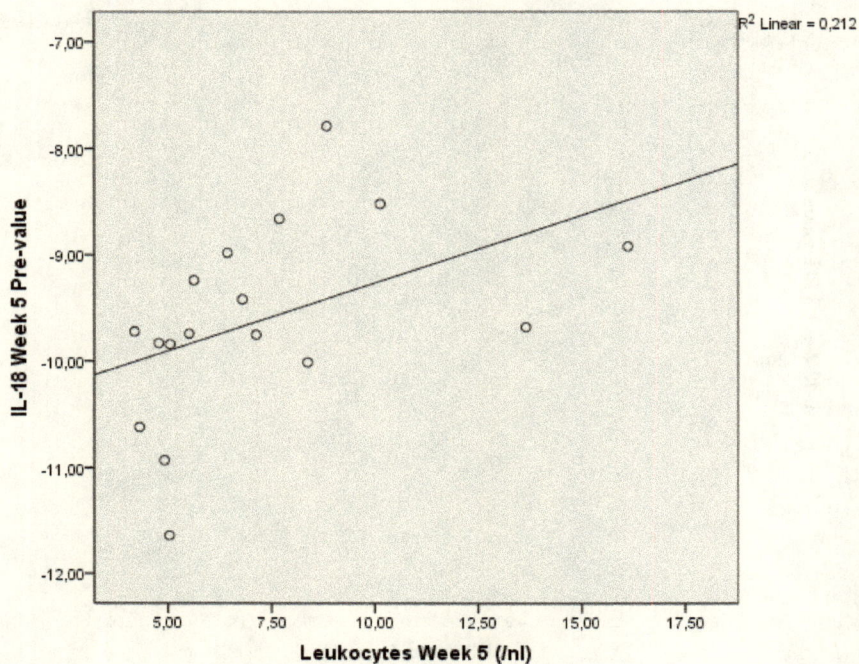

Figure 51: Scatter-plot: Correlation of Leukocytes (Week 5, /nl) and gene expression of IL-18 (Week 5, Pre-Value, Δ Ct)

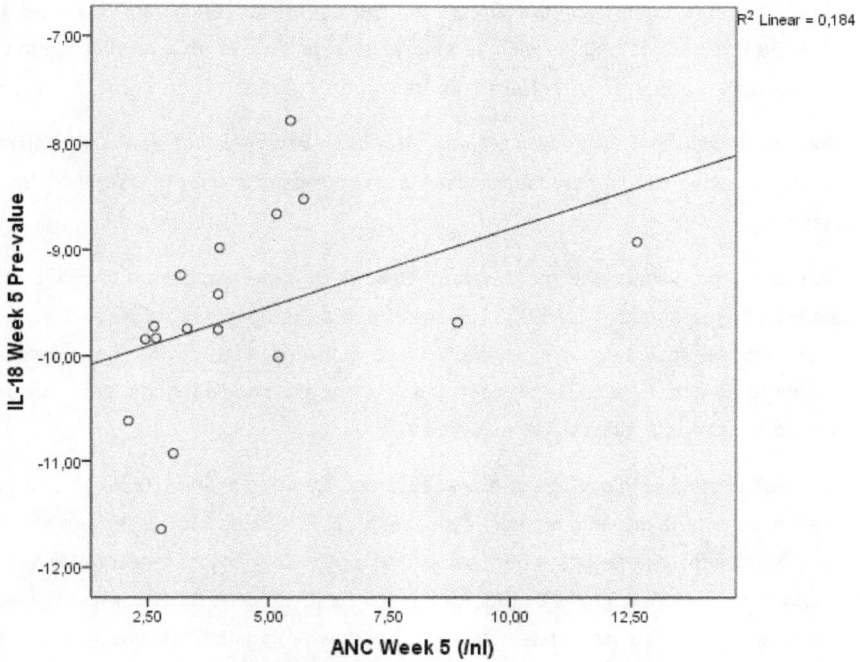

Figure 52: Scatter-plot: Correlation of ANC (Week 5, /nl) and gene expression of IL-18 (Week 5, Pre-Value, Δ Ct)

4.3.5 KINETICS OF GENE EXPRESSION PROFILING

In addition to correlation analysis, the kinetics of gene expression profiles was studied.

The use of Wilcoxon-test for paired samples showed that TNF is just temporary influenced by methotrexate with significant changes in medians between pre-values and 4-hour values at week 5 (p=0.035).

On the contrary, changes in the kinetics of other parameters such as FPGS, IL-6, IL-12A and IL-18 are of long duration and therefore seem to play an essential role in the mechanism of action of methotrexate in rheumatoid arthritis.

Pre-values taken before starting MTX therapy and mean values of week 5 (consisting of pre-values week 5, 4-hour values week 5 and pre-values week 6) were included in calculation.

Comparing pre-values and mean-values of week 5, gene expression of FPGS was statistically up-regulated (p=0.003), showing that polyglutamation of MTX is starting soon after the first drug administration. Once activated, the activity of this enzyme seems to be stable, because at week 5 no statistically significant changes were observed 4 hours after dosing (table 16 and 17).

Although in general relative gene-expression just tended to change (table 16 and 17), the kinetics of the pro-inflammatory cytokines IL-6, IL-12A and IL-18 showed statistically significant differences when comparing pre-values before starting MTX and mean-values of week 5 (p=0.011 for IL-6, 0.002 for IL-12A and 0.013 for IL-18). Gene expression of these parameters tend to be down-regulated. This may implicate MTX's effect against inflammatory conditions, mediated by IL-6, IL-12A and IL-18.

4.4 DISCUSSION

Using RT-PCR, the influence of methotrexate on the immune response of patients with rheumatoid arthritis was evaluated.

Gene expression analysis on mRNA level showed that methotrexate has a pleiotropic impact on the cytokine network, involved in the pathogenesis of rheumatoid arthritis.

Although in general relative gene-expression just tended to change (table 16 and 17), kinetics of the pro-inflammatory cytokines IL-6, IL-12A and IL-18 showed statistically significant differences when comparing pre-values before starting MTX and mean-values of week 5.

Higher C_{max} levels of erythrocyte MTXPG1 correlated with lower levels of the pro-inflammatory cytokines TNF, IL-6 and IL-12A, implicating that the accumulation of MTX in erythrocytes makes an important contribution to the anti-inflammatory effect of the drug.

Further, the impact of methotrexate on the gene expression of IL-18 shall be highlighted. Interestingly, a positive correlation of IL-18 with AUC levels of erythrocyte MTXPG1 and MTXPG2 as well as C_{max} levels of MTXPG2 and MTXPG3 was observed, meaning that a higher gene expression of IL-18 is linked to higher concentrations of MTXPG1 and MTXPG2. These results support the importance of MTX polyglutamates in drug response.

The findings are in accordance with Moeller and co-workers, who describe that the constitutive expression of IL-18 mRNA is significantly reduced in rheumatoid arthritis PBMCs [94]. The fact that IL-18 stimulates the production of IL-1ß and TNF in vitro and that IL-18 is enhanced in synovial tissues may be a possible explanation for this phenomenon. In addition,

The findings are confirmed by the fact that gene expression of TNF, IL-12A and IL-18 correlated with clinical parameters used in rheumatoid arthritis.

For TNF, a depressed gene expression accompanied by lower levels of monocytes was observed.

In addition, a lower gene expression of IL-12A correlated with a reduction in CRP and ANC.

Finally, IL-18 was shown to have a high impact on inflammatory parameters. So, a lower IL-18 gene expression involved a reduction in inflammatory parameters, such as ESR, leukocytes, CRP and ANC.

The power of MTX to down-regulate the expression of key cytokines such as TNF, IL-6, IL-12A and IL-18 is of particular interest to give some insights in its mode of pharmacological action in rheumatoid arthritis.

So the presented results extend the knowledge about the action of MTX. In previous studies [45, 95], MTX was shown to reduce IL-4, IL-6, IL-13 and TNF in whole blood cultures. The observation that IL-12A and IL-18 are additionally influenced by MTX broadens the understanding of the mechanism of action of the most widely used drug in rheumatoid arthritis.

However, it should be noted that patients were allowed to take concomitant corticosteroids to prevent disease progression. To eliminate this confounding factor, additional subgroup analyses for study participants taking methotrexate without concomitant corticosteroids are required.

5 SUMMARIZING DISCUSSION

Methotrexate is a cornerstone in the therapy of rheumatoid arthritis. Despite its long-lasting use, some questions concerning clinical practice remained open over several decades.

First of all, there was controversial discussion if methotrexate polyglutamates play an essential role in drug response and if their concentration may serve as potential marker for the efficacy of methotrexate.

Secondly, it was not well established if methotrexate should be started using conventional doses up to 15 mg per week or immediately at higher doses to accelerate clinical response.

Further, the large inter-patient variability in bioavailability (13-76% range) after oral administration consistently leads to clinically relevant discussions if methotrexate should be administered as oral or subcutaneous dose.

To clarify these questions and to increase knowledge about the mode of action of methotrexate in rheumatoid arthritis, the study presented in the thesis project at hand was designed.

A randomized, double-blinded, controlled clinical trial phase 4 including nineteen patients was performed in accordance with GCP guidelines and ethical principles that have their origin in the Declaration of Helsinki.

The primary project aims were to investigate the correlation of methotrexate polyglutamate concentrations with clinical response and to compare the efficacy of a conventional starting dose with a higher starting dose.

In addition, real time PCR was performed to evaluate the impact of methotrexate on the gene expression of selected pro-inflammatory cytokines (TNF, IL-6, IL-12A, IL-

17A and IL-18) and enzymes being involved in the metabolism of the drug (GGH, FPGS) in rheumatoid arthritis patients.

For pharmacokinetic analysis, plasma MTX and 7-OH-MTX as well as erythrocyte polyglutamates were measured by the use and optimization of two previously published HPLC methods [39, 77]. The distribution of MTX between plasma and erythrocytes – two different pharmacokinetic compartments – was described by the combined use of these approaches.

In erythrocytes, MTXPG1 occurred within 1.5 hours after drug administration. Even though plasma MTX was totally excreted by the kidneys within 48 hours, a redistribution of MTXPG1 to plasma MTX was observed 168 hours after MTX intake but before the second drug administration. This interesting phenomenon may be explained by a saturation mechanism of erythrocytes.

In general, the formation of MTXPG2 and MTXPG3 started within 168 hours after MTX intake. Steady-state of MTXPG1-3 was not achieved before week 10.

Supplementary to existing theories, pharmacokinetic-pharmacodynamic modeling identified *MTXPG2* as a potential marker for clinical outcome in rheumatoid arthritis. Higher levels of MTXPG2 went along with a significant reduction of DAS-28 at the end of the clinical trial at week 16. DAS-28 calculation incorporates clinical parameters (ESR, swollen and tender joints) as well as subjective parameters (VAS pain). Further, a negative correlation between C_{max} levels of MTXPG2 and eosinophils was observed, at week 10 even a negative correlation with basophils.

These correlations indicate a potential use of MTXPG2 in drug monitoring of MTX. Up to now, only long-chained polyglutamates were linked to a good MTX response.

Of clinical interest is the large inter- and intrapatient variability of methotrexate observed in the study collective. In some cases, subcutaneous administration of MTX resulted in higher MTX and polyglutamate levels. In contrast, other patients achieved higher concentrations after methotrexate given orally. As a consequence, subcutaneous administration of MTX did not result in a significant benefit to rheumatoid arthritis patients in the presented population.

To compare the pharmacokinetics of a higher starting dose and a standard dose, ten patients received a starting dose of 15 mg per week. Dose was escalated every two weeks until 25 mg per week. The second group (nine patients) started immediately with 25 mg MTX given orally once a week.

Performing HPLC analysis at week 1, C_{max}-levels of MTX and MTXPG1 were significantly higher in patients receiving the higher starting dose of 25 mg MTX per week.

However, the difference in pharmacokinetics was not relevant for clinical outcome, because a higher starting dose of MTX did not accelerate clinical improvement compared to a standard dose.

Potential limits of the pharmacokinetic analysis were interferences at the chromatographic positions of MTXPG4 and MTXPG5. As a consequence, these polyglutamates were not included in data analysis. Performing co-chromatography, these interferences were identified as polyglutamate 4 and polyglutamate 5. By the use of hydrolysis, PG4 and PG5 were metabolized to a shorter-chained polyglutamate resulting in an extra peak. This experiment may prove the natural occurrence of PG4 and PG5 in humans and subsequently relativizes the importance as potential outcome parameters in rheumatoid arthritis. For verification, further investigations are needed.

Using RT-PCR, the influence of methotrexate on the immune response of patients with rheumatoid arthritis was evaluated and a pharmacokinetic-pharmacodynamic-pharmacogenomic model was established.

Gene expression analysis on mRNA level showed, that methotrexate has a pleiotropic impact on the cytokine network involved in the pathogenesis of rheumatoid arthritis.

Although in general gene-expression just tended to change, the kinetics of the pro-inflammatory cytokines IL-6, IL-12A and IL-18 showed statistically significant differences comparing pre-values before MTX start and mean-values of week 5.

Higher C_{max} levels of erythrocyte MTXPG1 correlated with lower levels of the pro-inflammatory cytokines TNF, IL-6 and IL-12A, implicating that the accumulation of MTX in erythrocytes may contribute to the anti-inflammatory effect of the drug.

These findings are confirmed by the fact that the gene expression of TNF, IL-12A and IL-18 significantly correlated with clinical parameters used in rheumatoid arthritis. A depressed gene expression of TNF was accompanied by lower levels of monocytes. In addition, a lower gene expression of IL-12A correlated with a reduction in CRP and ANC.

Drug administration statistically significant reduced important clinical and subjective parameters such as DAS-28, HAQ-Score, VAS pain, VAS fatigue as well as PGA and EGA. In contrast, ESR was hardly reduced by the use of methotrexate. Other inflammatory parameters such as the CRP showed a trend towards a reduction, which was because of the limited sample size not of significance.

The original consideration, that a higher starting dose of MTX possibly accelerates clinical response to a higher extent than a standard dose, did not prove true. Although no difference in side effects was observed, a starting dose of 15 mg per week should be recommended to prevent potential impairment in liver and kidney function. In addition to the missing therapeutic benefit, the lower costs for a standard dose could be considered in making therapeutic decisions.

Supplemental to existing results, MTXPG2 - a short-chain polyglutamate - was found to correlate with important clinical parameters and is therefore a potential marker for clinical outcome in the therapy of rheumatoid arthritis.

Moreover, the power of MTX to modulate key cytokines such as TNF, IL-6, IL-12A and IL-18 is of particular interest and provides some insights into its mode of pharmacological action in rheumatoid arthritis.

The presented results extend the knowledge about the molecular action of MTX. In previous studies [95] MTX was shown to reduce IL-4, IL-6, IL-13 and TNF in whole blood cultures. The observation that IL-12A and IL-18 are influenced by MTX broadens the understanding of the mechanism of action of the most widely used drug in rheumatoid arthritis.

However, additional subgroup analyses for study participants taking methotrexate without concomitant corticosteroids or NSARs are required to clarify if MTX's effect is masked by the co-administration of other anti-inflammatory drugs.

6 CONCLUSION

Methotrexate is a mainstay in the therapy of rheumatoid arthritis, not least due to its positive benefit-risk-ratio.

Despite its long lasting use, some questions including metabolism, mode of administration, starting dose and mode of action remained open or are controversially discussed.

The presented randomized, double-blinded controlled clinical trial was designed to establish a pharmacokinetic-pharmacodynamic-pharmacogenomic model of methotrexate in rheumatoid arthritis.

It was shown, that the accumulation of methotrexate polyglutamates in erythrocytes has an impact on drug efficacy. MTXPG2 was identified as a potential marker for clinical outcome in rheumatoid arthritis with a positive correlation of MTXPG2 concentration and improvement in DAS-28, indicating a potential role of MTXPG2 in drug monitoring of MTX.

To establish an appropriate model to combine pharmacokinetics, pharmacodynamics and pharmacogenomics, gene expression analysis using RT-PCR was performed to evaluate the influence of methotrexate on the immune response of patients with rheumatoid arthritis.

Modeling of pharmacokinetics and gene expression showed, that the pro-inflammatory cytokines TNF, IL-6, IL-12A and IL-18 are influenced by methotrexate polyglutamates, implicating that drug accumulation in erythrocytes likely contributes to the anti-inflammatory effect of the drug.

Further, the pharmacodynamics of methotrexate significantly correlated with gene expression of TNF, IL-12A and IL-18, represented by a reduction of laboratory parameters used in rheumatoid arthritis.

In previous studies MTX was shown to reduce IL-4, IL-6, IL-13 and TNF in whole blood cultures [95]. Demonstrating that IL-12A and IL-18 are influenced by MTX in addition to the mentioned cytokines, the presented work broadens the understanding of the mechanism of action of the most widely used drug in rheumatoid arthritis and gives some more insight into its mode of pharmacological action.

Potential limits of the study are the proportionally small sample size and HPLC interferences, which were observed at the chromatographic positions of MTXPG4 and MTXPG5. Further, patients were allowed to take concomitant medications as corticosteroids and Non-steroidal Anti-Rheumatic Drugs (NSARs), which may influence the pharmacokinetics of methotrexate.

To conclude, methotrexate was shown to be a potent drug in the treatment of rheumatoid arthritis with a favorable benefit-risk ratio. Measurement of laboratory and clinical parameters at the end of the study demonstrated that MTX reduced DAS-28, HAQ-Score, PGA, EGA, VAS pain, VAS fatigue as well as the number of swollen and tender joints and the duration of morning stiffness.

As recommendation for clinical practice, methotrexate-based therapy should be started with a dose of 15 mg per week. Although no higher incidence of side effects was observed using 25 mg per week, a therapeutic benefit compared to a standard dose was missing. Further, a potential impairment in hepatic and renal function should be considered when using "high-dose" methotrexate.

For a better handling in clinical routine and due to a lack of benefit of subcutaneous administration, in general MTX should be started as oral dose. In individual cases, for example in patients with gastrointestinal side effects or insufficient therapeutic response, outcome may be improved by switching to s.c. administration.

To improve therapy and select patients not responding to MTX in time, the measurement of MTX serum and erythrocyte concentrations could be implemented in clinical routine. In particular, MTXPG2 seems to be a potential indicator for clinical response and may serve as a marker for drug monitoring.

7 APPENDICES

7.1 LIST OF ABBREVIATIONS

#	Number
%	Percent
°C	Degree Celsius
µl	Microliter
ABC	ATP-Binding Cassette
ACN	Acetonitrile
ACR	American College of Rheumatology
ADS	Alkyl-Diol Silica
AICAR	5-Aminoimidazole-4-Carboxamide Ribonucleotide
ALAT	Alanine Aminotransferase
AMP	Adenosine Monophosphate
ANC	Absolute Neutrophil Count
Anti-CCP	Anti-Cyclic Citrullinated Peptide
ASAT	Aspartate Aminotransferase
ATIC	5-Aminoimidazole-4-Imidazole Carboxamide Ribonucleotide Transformylase
AUC	Area Under the Curve
B (- cell)	Bursa of Fabricius
Bp	Base pair(s)
C	Carbon
CD	Cluster of Differentiation
cDNA	Complementary DNA
CI	Confidence Interval
Cm	Centimeter
C_{max}	Highest drug concentration observed

CNS	Central Nervous System
Conc.	Concentration
CRP	C-Reactive Protein
CV	Coefficient of Variation
DAS	Disease Activity Score
dATP	Deoxyadenosine Triphosphate
dCTP	Deoxycytidine Triphosphate
DEPC	Diethylpyrocarbonate
dGTP	Deoxyguanosine Triphosphate
DHF	Dihydrofolate
DHFR	Dihydrofolate Reductase
DI	Deciliter
DMARD	Disease-Modifying Antirheumatic Drug
DNA	Deoxyribonucleic Acid
dNTP	Deoxyribonucleotide Triphosphate
dTTP	Deoxythymidine Triphosphate
EDTA	Ethylendiaminetetraacetic
EGA	Evaluator Global Assessment
ESR	Erythrocyte Sedimentation Rate
et al.	Et alia
F	Female
Fc	Fragment crystalline
FPGS	Folylpolyglutamate Synthetase
FR	Folate Receptor
G	Gram
GAPDH	Glyceraldehyde-3-phosphate dehydrogenase
GCP	Good Clinical Practice
GGH	Gamma-glutamyl Hydrolase
GM-CSF	Granulocyte Macrophage – Colony Stimulating Factor
H	Hour
H_2O	Water
H_2O_2	Hydrogen Peroxide
HAQ	Health Assessment Questionnaire

HIV	Human Immunodeficiency Virus
HLA	Human Leukocyte Antigen
HPLC	High Pressure Liquid Chromatography
i.d.	Inner diameter
i.e.	In example
i.m.	Intramuscular
ICAM	Intracellular Adhesion Molecule
IFN	Interferon
IL	Interleukin
IL-R	Interleukin-Receptor
IUPAC	International Union of Pure and Applied Chemistry
Kd	Kilodalton
Kd	Kilodalton
Kg	Kilogram
L	Liter
LU*s	Luminescence Units per second
M	Male
m^2	Square meter
Mg	Milligram
$MgCl_2$	Magnesium Chloride
MHC	Major Histocompatibility Complex
Min	Minute
Mm	Millimeter
mM	Millimolar
mRNA	Messenger Ribonucleic Acid
MRP	Multidrug Resistance Protein
MTHFR	N^5,N^{10}-Methylentetrahydrofolate Reductase
MTX	Methotrexate
MTXPG	Methotrexate Polyglutamate
MW	Molecular Weight
NF-κB	Nuclear Factor- κB
NK cell	Natural Killer cell
Nl	Nanoliter

Nm	Nanometer
nM	Nanomolar
NSAR	Non-Steroidal Antirheumatic Drug
o.d.	Outer diameter
OH	Hydroxy
P	Probability
p.a.	Pro analysi
p.o.	Per os
PBMCs	Peripheral Blood Mononuclear Cells
PCR	Polymerase Chain Reaction
PGA	Patient Global Assessment
pH	Potentia Hydrogenii
pos.	Positive
R	Correlation Coefficient
r	Radius (mm)
R^2	Coefficient of Determination
RA	Rheumatoid Arthritis
RBC	Red Blood Cell
RCF	Relative Centrifugal Force
RFC	Reduced Folate Carrier
RNA	Ribonucleic Acid
RP	Reversed Phase
RPM	Revolutions Per Minute
RT	Reverse Transcriptase
RT-PCR	Real time-Polymerase Chain Reaction
s.c.	Subcutaneous
SD	Standard Deviation
SDS	Sodium Dodecyl Sulfate
SLC	Solute Carrier
SNP	Single Nucleotide Polymorphism
SW	Swollen
T	Time
T (- cell)	Thymus

TBAH	Tetrabutylammonium
TBE	Tris/Borate/EDTA
TEN	Tender
Th cell	T helper cell
THF	Tetrahydrofolate
T_{max}	Time at which the highest drug concentration occurs
TNF	Tumor Necrosis Factor
TYMS	Thymidylate Synthase
U	Unit
USA	United States of America
UV	Ultraviolet
VAS	Visual Analog Scale
VCAM	Vascular Cell Adhesion Molecule
Yr	Year

7.2 LIST OF TABLES

7.3 LIST OF FIGURES

12A

7.4 LABORATORY EQUIPMENT

ABI PRISM 7700 Sequence Detector

Agilent 1100 HPLC Chemstation system

Agilent Technologies Clear Wide Opening Crimp Vials 2 ml

Agilent Technologies Slvr Al Crmp Cap 11 mm

Bransonic 220 Ultrasonic Bath

Corning Bottle Top Filter W/45mm Neck, 0.22 µm CA, 500 ml

Corning Centrifuge Tubes 15 ml

Eppendorf Thermomixer Comfort

Falcon Pipettes

Gel Chamber (MWG, Biotech)

Gilson Pipettes

Gilson Pump 305

Graduent Block PCR express (Thermo electron corporation)

Hettich Centrifuge EBA 12

Hettich Rotanta 46 RSC

Hettich Universal 30 RF Table centrifuge

Hitachi U-2900 Spectrophotometer

Labinco L 24 Vortexer

Micro centrifuge (Harmony)

Micro tubes 1.5 ml (Sarstedt)

Millipore Filter HVHP 0.45 µm

Millipore Filter HVLP 0.45 µm

PCR Softubes 0.5 ml (Biozym)

pH Electrode (Metrohm)

pH Meter PHM 83 AUTOCAL (Radiometer)

Photochemical Reactor Aura Industries

Pipetus Pipette Controller

Sartorius BP 2100S Precision Balance

Sartorius Sterile Filtration Units

VWR Pasteur Pipettes

7.5 SOFTWARE

EndNote X2

Kinetica 2000

PASW Statistics 18

8 REFERENCES

1. Rindfleisch, J.A. and D. Muller, Diagnosis and management of rheumatoid arthritis. Am Fam Physician, 2005. 72(6): p. 1037-47.

2. Furst, D.E., et al., Tumor necrosis factor antagonists: different kinetics and/or mechanisms of action may explain differences in the risk for developing granulomatous infection. Semin Arthritis Rheum, 2006. 36(3): p. 159-67.

3. Sokka, T., Work disability in early rheumatoid arthritis. Clin Exp Rheumatol, 2003. 21(5 Suppl 31): p. S71-4.

4. Lefevre, S., et al., Synovial fibroblasts spread rheumatoid arthritis to unaffected joints. Nat Med, 2009. 15(12): p. 1414-1420.

5. Huber, L.C., et al., Synovial fibroblasts: key players in rheumatoid arthritis. Rheumatology (Oxford), 2006. 45(6): p. 669-75.

6. Firestein, G.S., Evolving concepts of rheumatoid arthritis. Nature, 2003. 423(6937): p. 356-361.

7. Goldblatt, F. and D.A. Isenberg, New therapies for rheumatoid arthritis. Clin Exp Immunol, 2005. 140(2): p. 195-204.

8. Neumann, E., et al., Local production of complement proteins in rheumatoid arthritis synovium. Arthritis Rheum, 2002. 46(4): p. 934-45.

9. Westwood, O.M., P.N. Nelson, and F.C. Hay, Rheumatoid factors: what's new? Rheumatology (Oxford), 2006. 45(4): p. 379-85.

10. Stern, L.J., et al., Crystal structure of the human class II MHC protein HLA-DR1 complexed with an influenza virus peptide. Nature, 1994. 368(6468): p. 215-221.

11. Weyand, C.M. and J.J. Goronzy, Association of MHC and rheumatoid arthritis. HLA polymorphisms in phenotypic variants of rheumatoid arthritis. Arthritis Res, 2000. 2(3): p. 212-6.

12. O'Dell, J.R., et al., HLA-DRB1 typing in rheumatoid arthritis: predicting response to specific treatments. Ann Rheum Dis, 1998. 57(4): p. 209-13.

13. Kerlan-Candon, S., et al., HLA-DRB1 gene transcripts in rheumatoid arthritis. Clin Exp Immunol, 2001. 124(1): p. 142-9.

14. Firestein, G.S., J.M. Alvaro-Gracia, and R. Maki, Quantitative analysis of cytokine gene expression in rheumatoid arthritis. J Immunol, 1990. 144(9): p. 3347-53.

15. Isomaki, P. and J. Punnonen, Pro- and anti-inflammatory cytokines in rheumatoid arthritis. Ann Med, 1997. 29(6): p. 499-507.

16. Kapral, T., et al., Methotrexate in rheumatoid arthritis is frequently effective, even if re-employed after a previous failure. Arthritis Res Ther, 2006. 8(2): p. R46.

17. van der Heijden, J.W., et al., Drug Insight: resistance to methotrexate and other disease-modifying antirheumatic drugs--from bench to bedside. Nat Clin Pract Rheumatol, 2007. 3(1): p. 26-34.

18. Miller, D.R., A tribute to Sidney Farber-- the father of modern chemotherapy. Br J Haematol, 2006. 134(1): p. 20-6.

19. Boehme, S.A. and M.J. Lenardo, Propriocidal apoptosis of mature T lymphocytes occurs at S phase of the cell cycle. European Journal of Immunology, 1993. 23(7): p. 1552-1560.

20. Chabner, B.A. and R.C. Young, Threshold Methotrexate Concentration for In Vivo Inhibition of DNA Synthesis in Normal and Tumorous Target Tissues. The Journal of Clinical Investigation, 1973. 52(8): p. 1804-1811.

21. Weinblatt, M.E., et al., Efficacy of low-dose methotrexate in rheumatoid arthritis. N Engl J Med, 1985. 312(13): p. 818-22.

22. Pincus, T., et al., Methotrexate as the "anchor drug" for the treatment of early rheumatoid arthritis. Clin Exp Rheumatol, 2003. 21(5 Suppl 31): p. S179-85.

23. Rau, R. and G. Herborn, Benefit and risk of methotrexate treatment in rheumatoid arthritis. Clin Exp Rheumatol, 2004. 22(5 Suppl 35): p. S83-94.

24. Pincus, T., et al., Evidence from clinical trials and long-term observational studies that disease-modifying anti-rheumatic drugs slow radiographic progression in rheumatoid arthritis: updating a 1983 review. Rheumatology (Oxford), 2002. 41(12): p. 1346-56.

25. Weinblatt, M.E., et al., Long-term prospective trial of low-dose methotrexate in rheumatoid arthritis. Arthritis Rheum, 1988. 31(2): p. 167-75.

26. Strand, V., et al., Treatment of active rheumatoid arthritis with leflunomide compared with placebo and methotrexate. Leflunomide Rheumatoid Arthritis Investigators Group. Arch Intern Med, 1999. 159(21): p. 2542-50.

27. Bathon, J.M., et al., A Comparison of Etanercept and Methotrexate in Patients with Early Rheumatoid Arthritis. N Engl J Med, 2000. 343(22): p. 1586-1593.

28. Bannwarth, B., et al., Clinical pharmacokinetics of low-dose pulse methotrexate in rheumatoid arthritis. Clin Pharmacokinet, 1996. 30(3): p. 194-210.

29. Angelis-Stoforidis, P., F.J. Vajda, and N. Christophidis, Methotrexate polyglutamate levels in circulating erythrocytes and polymorphs correlate with clinical efficacy in rheumatoid arthritis. Clin Exp Rheumatol, 1999. 17(3): p. 313-20.

30. Alarcon, G.S., I.C. Tracy, and W.D. Blackburn, Jr., Methotrexate in rheumatoid arthritis. Toxic effects as the major factor in limiting long-term treatment. Arthritis Rheum, 1989. 32(6): p. 671-6.

31. Prashker, M.J. and R.F. Meenan, The total costs of drug therapy for rheumatoid arthritis. A model based on costs of drug, monitoring, and toxicity. Arthritis Rheum, 1995. 38(3): p. 318-25.

32. Hamilton, R.A. and J.M. Kremer, Why intramuscular methotrexate may be more efficacious than oral dosing in patients with rheumatoid arthritis. Br J Rheumatol, 1997. 36(1): p. 86-90.

33. Tian, H. and B.N. Cronstein, Understanding the mechanisms of action of methotrexate: implications for the treatment of rheumatoid arthritis. Bull NYU Hosp Jt Dis, 2007. 65(3): p. 168-73.

34. Nakashima-Matsushita, N., et al., Selective expression of folate receptor beta and its possible role in methotrexate transport in synovial macrophages from patients with rheumatoid arthritis. Arthritis Rheum, 1999. 42(8): p. 1609-16.

35. Zeng, H., et al., Transport of methotrexate (MTX) and folates by multidrug resistance protein (MRP) 3 and MRP1: effect of polyglutamylation on MTX transport. Cancer Res, 2001. 61(19): p. 7225-32.

36. Galivan, J., Evidence for the cytotoxic activity of polyglutamate derivatives of methotrexate. Mol Pharmacol, 1980. 17(1): p. 105-10.

37. van Ede, A.E., et al., Methotrexate in rheumatoid arthritis: an update with focus on mechanisms involved in toxicity. Semin Arthritis Rheum, 1998. 27(5): p. 277-92.

38. Szeto, D.W., et al., Human thymidylate synthetase--III : Effects of methotrexate and folate analogs. Biochemical Pharmacology, 1979. 28(17): p. 2633-2637.

39. Dervieux, T., et al., HPLC determination of erythrocyte methotrexate polyglutamates after low-dose methotrexate therapy in patients with rheumatoid arthritis. Clin Chem, 2003. 49(10): p. 1632-41.

40. Cronstein, B.N., et al., Methotrexate inhibits neutrophil function by stimulating adenosine release from connective tissue cells. Proc Natl Acad Sci U S A, 1991. 88(6): p. 2441-5.

41. Baggott, J.E., et al., Antifolates in rheumatoid arthritis: a hypothetical mechanism of action. Clin Exp Rheumatol, 1993. 11 Suppl 8: p. S101-5.

42. Gruber, H.E., et al., Increased adenosine concentration in blood from ischemic myocardium by AICA riboside. Effects on flow, granulocytes, and injury. Circulation, 1989. 80(5): p. 1400-11.

43. Cronstein, B.N., THE MECHANISM OF ACTION OF METHOTREXATE. Rheumatic Disease Clinics of North America, 1997. 23(4): p. 739-755.

44. Cutolo, M., et al., Anti-inflammatory mechanisms of methotrexate in rheumatoid arthritis. Ann Rheum Dis, 2001. 60(8): p. 729-35.

45. Gerards, A.H., et al., Inhibition of cytokine production by methotrexate. Studies in healthy volunteers and patients with rheumatoid arthritis. Rheumatology (Oxford), 2003. 42(10): p. 1189-96.

46. Seitz, M., M. Zwicker, and P. Loetscher, Effects of methotrexate on differentiation of monocytes and production of cytokine inhibitors by monocytes. Arthritis Rheum, 1998. 41(11): p. 2032-8.

47. Montesinos, M.C., et al., Reversal of the antiinflammatory effects of methotrexate by the nonselective adenosine receptor antagonists theophylline and caffeine: evidence that the antiinflammatory effects of methotrexate are mediated via multiple adenosine receptors in rat adjuvant arthritis. Arthritis Rheum, 2000. 43(3): p. 656-63.

48. Nesher, G., M. Mates, and S. Zevin, Effect of caffeine consumption on efficacy of methotrexate in rheumatoid arthritis. Arthritis Rheum, 2003. 48(2): p. 571-2.

49. Morgan, S.L., et al., Supplementation with folic acid during methotrexate therapy for rheumatoid arthritis. A double-blind, placebo-controlled trial. Ann Intern Med, 1994. 121(11): p. 833-41.

50. Slot, O., Changes in plasma homocysteine in arthritis patients starting treatment with low-dose methotrexate subsequently supplemented with folic acid. Scand J Rheumatol, 2001. 30(5): p. 305-7.

51. Lange, H., et al., Folate therapy and in-stent restenosis after coronary stenting. N Engl J Med, 2004. 350(26): p. 2673-81.

52. Matherly, L.H. and D.I. Goldman, Membrane transport of folates. Vitam Horm, 2003. 66: p. 403-56.

53. Rau Rolf, H.I., Hunzelmann Nicolas, Das Methotrexat-Buch. Aktuelle Therapiekonzepte in der Rheumatologie und Dermatologie. 2007, Bremen: Uni-Med.

54. Hoekstra, M., et al., Factors associated with toxicity, final dose, and efficacy of methotrexate in patients with rheumatoid arthritis. Ann Rheum Dis, 2003. 62(5): p. 423-6.

55. Kremer, J.M., et al., Methotrexate for rheumatoid arthritis. Suggested guidelines for monitoring liver toxicity. American College of Rheumatology. Arthritis Rheum, 1994. 37(3): p. 316-28.

56. Morgan, C., et al., Contribution of patient related differences to multidrug resistance in rheumatoid arthritis. Ann Rheum Dis, 2003. 62(1): p. 15-9.

57. Wood, A.J.J., et al., Intrinsic and Acquired Resistance to Methotrexate in Acute Leukemia. New England Journal of Medicine, 1996. 335(14): p. 1041-1048.

58. Bertino, J.R., et al., Resistance Mechanisms to Methotrexate in Tumors. Oncologist, 1996. 1(4): p. 223-226.

59. Rahman, P., D. Hefferton, and D. Robb, Increased MDR1 P-glycoprotein expression in methotrexate resistance: comment on the article by Yudoh et al. Arthritis Rheum, 2000. 43(7): p. 1661-2.

60. Norris, M.D., et al., Involvement of MDR1 P-glycoprotein in multifactorial resistance to methotrexate. Int J Cancer, 1996. 65(5): p. 613-9.

61. Stranzl, T., et al., Expression of folylpolyglutamyl synthetase predicts poor response to methotrexate therapy in patients with rheumatoid arthritis. Clin Exp Rheumatol, 2003. 21(1): p. 27-32.

62. Dervieux, T., et al., Polyglutamation of methotrexate with common polymorphisms in reduced folate carrier, aminoimidazole carboxamide ribonucleotide transformylase, and thymidylate synthase are associated with methotrexate effects in rheumatoid arthritis. Arthritis Rheum, 2004. 50(9): p. 2766-74.

63. Wessels, J.A., et al., Efficacy and toxicity of methotrexate in early rheumatoid arthritis are associated with single-nucleotide polymorphisms in genes coding for folate pathway enzymes. Arthritis Rheum, 2006. 54(4): p. 1087-95.

64. Hider, S.L., I.N. Bruce, and W. Thomson, The pharmacogenetics of methotrexate. Rheumatology (Oxford), 2007. 46(10): p. 1520-4.

65. Constantin, A., et al., Antiinflammatory and immunoregulatory action of methotrexate in the treatment of rheumatoid arthritis: evidence of increased interleukin-4 and interleukin-10 gene expression demonstrated in vitro by competitive reverse transcriptase-polymerase chain reaction. Arthritis Rheum, 1998. 41(1): p. 48-57.

66. Stamp, L.K., et al., Methotrexate polyglutamate concentrations are not associated with disease control in rheumatoid arthritis patients receiving long-term methotrexate therapy. Arthritis Rheum, 2010. 62(2): p. 359-68.

67. Schnabel, A., et al., Tolerability of methotrexate starting with 15 or 25 mg/week for rheumatoid arthritis. Rheumatol Int, 1994. 14(1): p. 33-8.

68. Lambert, C.M., et al., Dose escalation of parenteral methotrexate in active rheumatoid arthritis that has been unresponsive to conventional doses of methotrexate: a randomized, controlled trial. Arthritis Rheum, 2004. 50(2): p. 364-71.

69. Visser, K. and D. van der Heijde, Optimal dosage and route of administration of methotrexate in rheumatoid arthritis: a systematic review of the literature. Annals of the Rheumatic Diseases, 2009. 68(7): p. 1094-1099.

70. Braun, J., et al., Comparison of the clinical efficacy and safety of subcutaneous versus oral administration of methotrexate in patients with active rheumatoid arthritis: Results of a six-month, multicenter, randomized, double-blind, controlled, phase IV trial. Arthritis & Rheumatism, 2008. 58(1): p. 73-81.

71. Wegrzyn, J., P. Adeleine, and P. Miossec, Better efficacy of methotrexate given by intramuscular injection than orally in patients with rheumatoid arthritis. Ann Rheum Dis, 2004. 63(10): p. 1232-4.

72. Arnett, F.C., et al., The American Rheumatism Association 1987 revised criteria for the classification of rheumatoid arthritis. Arthritis Rheum, 1988. 31(3): p. 315-24.

73. Greenwood, M.C., D.V. Doyle, and M. Ensor, Does the Stanford Health Assessment Questionnaire have potential as a monitoring tool for subjects with rheumatoid arthritis? Ann Rheum Dis, 2001. 60(4): p. 344-8.

74. Cronstein, B.N., Low-Dose Methotrexate: A Mainstay in the Treatment of Rheumatoid Arthritis. Pharmacological Reviews, 2005. 57(2): p. 163-172.

75. Swierkot, J. and J. Szechinski, Methotrexate in rheumatoid arthritis. Pharmacol Rep, 2006. 58(4): p. 473-92.

76. Yu, Z. and D. Westerlund, Ion-pair chromatography of methotrexate in a column-switching system using an alkyl-diol silica precolumn for direct injection of plasma. J Chromatogr A, 1996. 742(1-2): p. 113-20.

77. Yu, Z., D. Westerlund, and K.S. Boos, Determination of methotrexate and its metabolite 7-hydroxymethotrexate by direct injection of human plasma into a column-switching liquid chromatographic system using post-column photochemical reaction with fluorimetric detection. J Chromatogr B Biomed Sci Appl, 1997. 689(2): p. 379-86.

78. Baeyens, W.R., et al., Application of an alkyl-diol silica precolumn in a column-switching system for the determination of meloxicam in plasma. J Pharm Biomed Anal, 2003. 32(4-5): p. 839-46.

79. Dalrymple, J.M., et al., Pharmacokinetics of oral methotrexate in patients with rheumatoid arthritis. Arthritis Rheum, 2008. 58(11): p. 3299-308.

80. Liote, F., et al., Blood monocyte activation in rheumatoid arthritis: increased monocyte adhesiveness, integrin expression, and cytokine release. Clin Exp Immunol, 1996. 106(1): p. 13-9.

81. Kubista, M., et al., The real-time polymerase chain reaction. Mol Aspects Med, 2006. 27(2-3): p. 95-125.

82. Galivan, J., et al., Glutamyl hydrolase. pharmacological role and enzymatic characterization. Pharmacol Ther, 2000. 85(3): p. 207-15.

83. Schneider, E. and T.J. Ryan, Gamma-glutamyl hydrolase and drug resistance. Clin Chim Acta, 2006. 374(1-2): p. 25-32.

84. Leclerc, G.J., et al., Analysis of folylpoly-gamma-glutamate synthetase gene expression in human B-precursor ALL and T-lineage ALL cells. BMC Cancer, 2006. 6: p. 132.

85. Choy, E.H. and G.S. Panayi, Cytokine pathways and joint inflammation in rheumatoid arthritis. N Engl J Med, 2001. 344(12): p. 907-16.

86. Schulze-Koops, H. and J.R. Kalden, The balance of Th1/Th2 cytokines in rheumatoid arthritis. Best Pract Res Clin Rheumatol, 2001. 15(5): p. 677-91.

87. McInnes, I.B. and G. Schett, Cytokines in the pathogenesis of rheumatoid arthritis. Nat Rev Immunol, 2007. 7(6): p. 429-442.

88. Hamza, T., J.B. Barnett, and B. Li, Interleukin 12 a key immunoregulatory cytokine in infection applications. Int J Mol Sci, 2010. 11(3): p. 789-806.

89. Kolls, J.K. and A. Linden, Interleukin-17 family members and inflammation. Immunity, 2004. 21(4): p. 467-76.

90. Yu, J.J. and S.L. Gaffen, Interleukin-17: a novel inflammatory cytokine that bridges innate and adaptive immunity. Front Biosci, 2008. 13: p. 170-7.

91. Hwang, S.Y., et al., IL-17 induces production of IL-6 and IL-8 in rheumatoid arthritis synovial fibroblasts via NF-kappaB- and PI3-kinase/Akt-dependent pathways. Arthritis Res Ther, 2004. 6(2): p. R120-8.

92. Gracie, J.A., et al., A proinflammatory role for IL-18 in rheumatoid arthritis. J Clin Invest, 1999. 104(10): p. 1393-401.

93. Gracie, J.A., S.E. Robertson, and I.B. McInnes, Interleukin-18. J Leukoc Biol, 2003. 73(2): p. 213-24.

94. Moller, B., et al., Expression of interleukin-18 and its monokine-directed function in rheumatoid arthritis. Rheumatology (Oxford), 2001. 40(3): p. 302-9.

95. Wessels, J.A., T.W. Huizinga, and H.J. Guchelaar, Recent insights in the pharmacological actions of methotrexate in the treatment of rheumatoid arthritis. Rheumatology (Oxford), 2008. 47(3): p. 249-55.

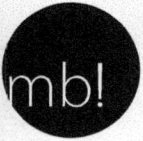

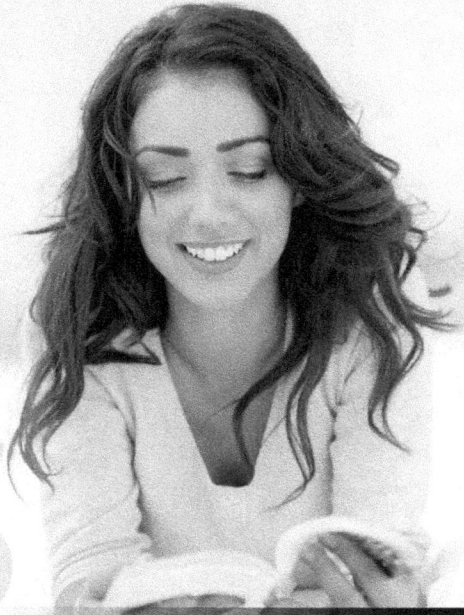

www.ingramcontent.com/pod-product-compliance
Lightning Source LLC
Chambersburg PA
CBHW02105721O326
41598CB00016B/1236